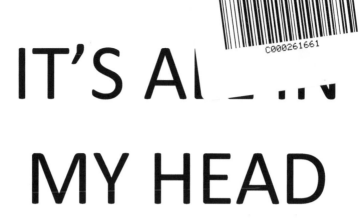

IT'S ALL IN MY HEAD

MY HEAD

How to Survive a Brain Tumour

and Find Peace of Mind

JO BARLOW

This book is dedicated to:

My Brain Tumour. Thank you for helping me understand that I can no longer let things 'do my head in' and showing me the many lessons I needed to learn in really being me and happy. You almost killed me but you saved me too. ♥

My husband Dave. Thank you for sitting and waiting outside the operating theatre for almost 6 hours and for telling me 'you did it' the minute I was wheeled through the doors. ♥ At that moment I knew I was safe and that you were, and always have been, here for me when I need it the most. ♥

My children- Adam, Zach, Calla and Roan. Thank you for dealing so well with what was a really tough 2016 and for looking after your totally sober, but very drunk, mother. ♥ If there is one thing I wish you to understand from this book- it's to always be you. Be proud of your amazing selves and your talents and don't ever give up on your dreams and joy. It's YOUR life, live it as you please.

My Mum and Dad. Above all thank you for paying for my MRI... things may have been very much different without it, and your support. I owe you my life in more ways than one! ♥

Mr Jones and all at St George's Hospital, Tooting. Thank you. ♥ Thank you for your skill and patience. ♥ And extra thanks for all the hand holding, listening to me crying, support, positivity and understanding. ♥

"We must see all scars as beauty.
Okay?
This will be our secret.
Because take it from me, a scar
does not form on the dying.
A scar means,
"I survived."

– From Little Bee: A novel, Chris Cleave

Contents

Introduction

This original idea for writing this book was from when I first knew I was having brain surgery, I looked online but could not see any book that felt it would give me the strength to help me overcome the huge fear and the many questions I had. So even then I decided if there weren't any, I would write one.

During my hospital stay I spoke to a couple of the nurses who also agreed there was nothing aimed at people who find hospitals and their machines, bleeps, and comments scary. The empaths who absorb every last emotion in the room.

I hope that my writing down how I felt both emotionally and the odd sensations that worried me will support and help others who have been diagnosed with a brain tumour and are needing surgery, as well as inform friends and family how they may feel and what may help them too.

I also hope that the total change in my belief system and realisations after will help anyone who is having to go through a health crisis or supporting a patient of any kind, that you can either look for the negative, or the positive in any situation.

Chapter 1 - Drunk on Water

"Ow...I don't think I should have done that." I have been painting around the edges of the ceiling in the lounge, stupidly holding my neck up as it was aching, but almost as soon as I put the paint brush down I start getting sharp pains in my neck. It is like someone was flicking an elastic band into my neck every so often and making me jolt. But thankfully the ceiling was now painted, the final bit of re-decorating the room, I just needed to put the kids items and decorations back on the shelves and I could rest. However, a week or so later the pains still haven't gone - they seem to have less of a sharpness yet last longer; so I go to the osteopath who tells me all seems ok with my spine and it should go in time, and gives me some muscle strengthening exercises to do once it has.

It's December 2015 and although I don't ever do much differently over Christmas than any other week of the winter, it still means I have to do some extra things, so I put on various types of scarf indoors to try and keep my neck warm; hopefully stopping the pains and get on with it. But each day I am getting a few sharp pains in my neck that don't seem to be going away and I don't feel I can turn my head as well as I could before. It feels wrong.

I'm driving and feel I'm tired, cannot concentrate and need to keep blinking to stop getting blurry vision – yet it's before lunchtime and I had a good night's sleep. Why does it feel so hard to think? I turn the music on to something that will inspire me, open the window for some fresh air and continue.

Ok, so I don't enjoy Christmas most years, but we are not doing much at all and I am not stressed about it at the moment, so why have I got this constant dull headache in what feels like the lump at the back of my head - the atlas joint? I don't even have headaches. I can count the number of times I have ever had a headache on one hand. And the neck pains are still not reducing, they are still shooting and making me jolt several times a day.

It's January. I am walking the dog on the footpath on the way to the park, but I feel wobbly, like I am not able to walk straight and my energy has been sucked out of me. If I look down as I walk I almost feel travel sick, like the ground is moving too fast. But I am walking.

My husband, Dave, is playing a gig at a pub. Why am I feeling so 'dizzy'? I feel like I could fall off the stool I am sitting on. Maybe I am detoxing or something? After all I am eating foods to help detox me right now. Maybe that is causing the dizziness? Maybe it was the vitamins I recently started that I am having a reaction to? After all I felt odd before when I was taking something similar.

A week or so later, I am walking up some stairs in a pub as we are at another gig. I am totally sober (I haven't drunk alcohol for well over 20 years) yet I feel drunk, like I cannot quite get my balance and coordinate the 'moving' steps as I walk up the stairs. My legs don't seem to be working right if I think about it. I hold on the handrail and get on with it. So, I'm dizzy, feeling drunk and still having neck pains. Great, now I am getting stressed and anxious too - that's really not helping the dizziness feel better. I want to cry and go home, yet instead I shut up and pretend I am OK. I can do that, I have done it many times before when I have panicked and felt ill, screaming inside yet smiling outwardly.

The dog and I are at the park. As I am walking I have the strangest sensation that my vision is like a home camera on a cheap TV show. Where my head, and with it my vision, are bouncing up and down as I walk, just as the camera would show if it was recorded in your hand, rather than the normal smooth walking movement where your eyes don't see any jolting.

Dave and Calla are away for a few days. I have to go on the bus to take my son to a Judo class, as I don't have a car. I feel I cannot coordinate a 'new task' and all the effort it is seeming to take to do anything, but still get there - although feeling more and more anxious by the minute. I sit in the school hall, where the Judo is being taught, feeling exhausted and terrified at the same time. I can't seem to focus right and still have this constant dizziness - although in varying degrees of severity. I sit and read a meditation e-book I had downloaded in the hope that I can somehow calm myself, but it's not working. I feel stressed up to my eyeballs! I feel I am having constant 'fight or flight' panic attacks daily. As we go home we are walking back down the road and I just feel my body is not connected to my brain... my legs are moving, but I don't know how. I want to go home and just sit down to rest. I feel almost sick as I am walking, but I have my child with me, so I just hold it all together, keep talking to him and silently sob inside. I get in, sit down for a minute, then cook dinner, eat and wash up, and then all but collapse on the sofa.

It's Dave's birthday. We go out for a meal. I feel I am so tired I cannot walk straight, but I'm not tired. I have to really concentrate that I am not crashing into other chairs, tables or people in the restaurant, yet I still don't seem to be able to totally manage it right and feel myself bouncing off things. I drop my coat, then my handbag. I can't pick them up easily. I have to concentrate not to make a mess and drop my food. My eyes are blinking and trying to focus better as my vision doesn't feel right. I just want to go home.

We go out to watch another band play at a pub, I walk to the toilet and bump into someone as he turned round - because I simply couldn't get out of the way in time. I then get a push in the back on my other side by his friend as I presume he thought I was either just pissed or did it on purpose... but I'm drinking water and I didn't 'try' to walk into him, I just couldn't move that quickly out of the way. Tears are starting to run down my face before I even get to the toilet door just a few steps away, and I just sit on the loo and cry. What's wrong with me? I stop myself, brush myself down, sort my face out, try and think positive thoughts (and that these two men are probably pissed themselves) and go back outside. Drinking my water!

Chapter 2 - Pain in the Neck

It's the 25th January. I was going to go out in the car to meet a friend, Alison, who was going to do a Bowen treatment on me, but feel too dizzy and scared to go as it is a thirty minute drive away and on main roads and there is no way I am able to manage that. Crying, I get Dave, and we book to see a doctor at my registered G.P. practice, Giggs Hill Surgery, instead.

Going to a doctor is a big thing as I don't do doctors or G.P's unless it's an emergency. I don't trust them ever since I was given antibiotics for acne as a teen...for 7 years! Especially as when after a couple of these years I developed bad Irritable Bowel Syndrome to the point I could barely eat as I had all but constant nausea and pain. I had tubes and camera's down my throat and was seen be several specialists. I had asked the doctors if the antibiotics and IBS were related and they all said 'no', the antibiotics only work on the skin and it couldn't possibly be the antibiotics causing the IBS, or any stomach problem.

However a few years later I found a nurses book with pharmaceutical drug/common medicine side effects and the very symptoms I had <u>were</u> listed as side effects of the antibiotic I was taking! Then when my wisdom teeth were removed a year or so after I stopped the antibiotics, my teeth were a lovely dark stain of orangey brown. Caused from the antibiotics staining them as they were growing. They are in fact so badly discoloured that the dentist kept the teeth as they were 'medically interesting' as an extreme example of how bad antibiotic staining can be. If antibiotics did this to my teeth, what did they do to my bones and rest of my body? I gave up with doctors and had to help myself and my IBS get sorted from diet, homeopathy and listening to my body. Many times since then I have disagreed with doctors seemingly 'take a harmless drug to fix that' belief, and it's even harder when they never respect my viewpoint, take my beliefs (often researched for a very long time) as wrong, ill-informed or not scientific, and therefore, stupid. Many a time have I 'agreed to disagree' and walked out saying it's my body and my choice.

I get to the G.P. surgery and see one of the locum doctors there, saying I have now been feeling dizzy most days for a few weeks. She gets me to do some coordination tests. I am fine with the moving my hand to my nose and back to her moving finger test, but I can barely walk straight. I try to do the 'drink drive test', where you walk touching your heel to toe in a straight line, and I simply cannot. I can't even get one heel and toe to touch together without wobbling over. I didn't realise I was this bad. I don't know whether to laugh or cry, but I am scared as to why I feel so awful. I ask the doctor 'does she think it's a brain tumour' and she said, no, it is very unlikely. But there is something massively up and it's either serious or acute, and I want to know what. She refers me for tests and a physiotherapist...

I post on Facebook that night:

> "Maybe if I started drinking I might walk straight?
>
> ...the joys of vertigo! ☹"

6th February. Written to a friend.

> "Oh and to top it off I damaged my neck when I painted the ceiling last year... After seeing osteopath, it has gradually got worse - pains and pounding... and seemingly with the dizziness, but I think they are 2 separate issues? But I still need to do something with my neck as if I bend down wrong it is horrendous ☹

I feel like I'm falling apart and totally depressed and anxious (I have seen that when your body gets dizzy you automatically put out fight or flight and so flood your body with adrenaline which doesn't help anxiety! ☹).

A couple of weeks later, despite my insane fears with each test - that this could be my problem and imagining all the worst case scenarios, my blood tests and heart scan are both normal. ENT appointment date is still not for another few weeks.

I book an opticians appointment, maybe my eyes are somehow causing these problems? But my eyes are fine, I do have a very slight prescription, but not enough to have to wear glasses for driving and nothing that would cause dizziness. Although oddly my prescription is opposite from the year before - the opposite eye is weaker. I get some glasses anyway in the hope that they will help my vision.

I am now consciously taking care when I turn around, bend down or walk past something so I don't crash into it or lose my balance. I feel I am walking with my arms out to balance me. When I am at a gig and carrying a full drink to Dave in a less known place than at home I have to carefully watch, think where I am going, and take careful steps so I won't spill the pint or trip over the wires on the floor. I have to stop and take deliberate moves when stepping around things or walking up a step.

I see a physiotherapist, who gives me some basic neck exercises to hopefully reduce the neck pain and with it stop the dizziness. She seems sure that I damaged my neck when painting, as it now clicks and grates - which means I have significant signs of arthritis in it. I tell her it didn't do this even a few months ago, but she just tells me it can suddenly come on.

26th February. I have the ENT appointment. Dave drives me to Epsom, we struggle to find the right area of the building as the letter really isn't clear, or my head can't comprehend it. It all feels really exhausting and I am getting more and more frustrated and grumpy. We arrive a few minutes late but get told its ok, so we wait for the appointment. Once again I am feeling a mix of wanting to get an answer and wanting to query any opinion the doctor may have. I have that feeling of dread where I will have to instantly know what may be helpful and what may be just an Elastoplast, or do more damage to my overall health. I can't back up my views if I have not heard of something before, but I know I probably won't agree if they want to give me a prescription. I feel I need a doctorate myself, so I know what to question and why. I also know they don't give you the option to come back and question them, and so many ridicule my views as they are not what most doctors believe.

I get called in and the doctor seems friendly - so I smile back cautiously, not daring to trust him yet. I get turned upside down a bit by him as he looks at my eyes to watch my response, and then gets me to stand up while shutting my eyes as he attempts to knock me over. He promises to catch me when I wobble, and does. He even requests a hearing test where I sit in a booth and record when I can hear sounds. I can hear them ok, but I have to shut my eyes as the booth is made from punched metal with circular gaps in it, and it is making my vision go insane as I cannot focus right. But it all shows as normal, that my hearing is really good and that the dizziness is clearly not caused by my ears. The consultant also cannot connect the neck pain in any way with my ears but suggests because of this and when it started, both him (and the other consultant in the clinic) think it could be a neck issue causing my problems. He also suggests that I could possibly be continuing or making worse an existing problem by being anxious about it. I agree and say it is very hard not to have a fight or flight response, when I can feel it happens each time I wobble and almost fall – which happens several times a day! I get told I should get my G.P. to refer me to either a neurologist or neurosurgeon, or possibly a rheumatologist - depending on who the consultants are in my area, but he will tell the G.P. this in a letter.

For the 29 days of February I have written down I have had 23 days of bad dizziness and 18 days with severe head pains, neck pounding or headache. Whatever it is - it's getting worse.

I am feeling so awful we book an emergency appointment with Giggs Hill, it is over the 10 days or so we were told the letter would take to arrive from the ENT department so I hope it has got there and they can refer me further. At this appointment I see Dr Vo from the practice, whom I have never seen before, and she asks why I am here. I can't walk properly (Dave has had to walk me into this appointment), I am constantly dizzy, I have pains in my head and neck that when I cough, sneeze or strain they feel worse, I am getting headaches at night and just don't feel right and feel uncoordinated. She doesn't seem concerned, does some basic tests (but not the drink drive one) and says all looks normal. I query could it be a brain tumour or something serious and she says no my neurological signs are all fine. I ask can I get referred to a neurologist, but I am told I cannot be referred yet as they have not received the details back from the ENT appointment suggesting this, plus I am not taking painkillers.

"Um…why would I take a pain killer that upsets my stomach and gives me nausea for something that only hurts on and off?"

"Well I can't refer you to a neurologist if we have not tried the basic treatments. I can offer you diazepam instead- would you like to try that?"

As I look incredulously at her thinking 'Why on earth would you offer me valium? Isn't that banned yet?'

I say "No thank you, I don't need drugging, I've had diazepam briefly before and it spaces me out"

She tut's and rolls her eyes at me. I am just sitting in total disbelief as to what she has just offered me, and feel I am justified in thinking many doctors are insane!

So ... as I apparently need to take something to relieve the pain (rather than address it) I end up accepting ibuprofen gel to put directly on my neck which I need to try for at least a week.

As I go to leave she makes it clear that this was an emergency appointment, so she only has so much time to discuss things, but as mine is a chronic problem I would need to book any further appointments as 'routine' and not the 'emergency' (booked on the day) appointments. She tells me that emergency is only for things such as sudden infections.

It takes me two days to decide to use the gel as I just don't want to cover up the pain and not sort out the actual problem. I am torn with this standard medical approach and what they call a benign drug, against my belief that we are not born paracetamol or ibuprofen deficient- so why would I take it and risk upsetting my body further? How is it supposed help with the dizziness? Plus it's not like the pain is continuous and I can't cope with it.

In the end I decide I will use the gel in the hope it will either relax my neck enough to heal whatever is causing the problem, or I can get a neurologist referral if it doesn't help - which I apparently can't get without using something for pain relief. And, well, the movement in my neck is getting worse by the day.

1st March. Written to a friend – who I had already discussed feeling dizzy and having neck pain with previously.

> "Any ideas? It has never fully gone away since November - each day I either have sharp pain in neck to head, pounding when I get up or down, or look up, a general stiff neck where I cannot turn well, as well as grinding in neck joint. I also have been getting dizziness / off balance. I failed miserably at the walking in a straight line test.
> I have seen GP, been seen by ENT and physio (only last week but it seems to be worse since - but possibly just as hormonal?) had blood and echocardiogram/ECG tests and all 'normal'.
> The ENT guy did say he was going to ask GP to refer me to neurologist or back surgeon etc (whatever we have in this area) as he was sure it was down to neck damage too.
> Any ideas? From wacky to standard? Or know of an emotional cause? x thank you x"

Dave is playing at another gig, I am sitting on a low stool by a table with another stool in a row right next to it. I move over onto the second one to let a friend sit down in the seat where I was sitting and promptly tip the stool up - as I follow with it. I feel myself falling in slow motion as I try to put my hand to the floor to stop myself. But, oh no, this gives way too. So I end up face first totally flat on the floor, hitting my thigh really badly on the fireplace edging, just missing my face and head on the other items in the fireplace whilst feeling like a drunken idiot. Which is slightly ironic as I am still drinking water and probably the only person in the pub not to have drunk any alcohol! I've scared Dave, as all he could see was me suddenly spread on the floor. I get some Homeopathic aconite for him, some arnica for me and go stop myself from crying in the toilet, especially as I see the lump and bruise already appearing on my leg. I come back, sit down and suddenly want to bawl my eyes out as the shock hits me.

I am sure I didn't pass out, but it feels like something happened as to why I couldn't stop myself. I feel so stupid and just want to cry. All the negative fears I have had in my life want to come up for me to cry over - they all need releasing with this shock. Later that night I get a nice big black bruise on my thigh, which progresses to a lovely green, yellow and purple bruise with lines in it- the same width apart as the lines in the decorative fireplace bricks!

9th March. The third doctor appointment I had booked long before the emergency appointment last time. It is again with Dr Vo - the same G.P who I saw last. This time she says I will need to have a neck x-ray before she will consider referring me, "As after all a neurologist will only insist on one anyway".

So therefore I need the x-ray done to see if that finds a problem the G.P. can rule out first, before I get a referral. As I leave the surgery I book another doctor appointment for when the G.P. estimates the x-ray results should be back in 2-3 weeks. I get an appointment for the 29th March which was also the earliest they could do!

I really need to do something for my head and neck, I need to see someone who can help, and right now I can't see any other option but to follow the system. So I reluctantly go straight to the local clinic and get the x-ray. I wouldn't normally just have an x-ray unless I felt there was a good reason - which I don't - and bearing in mind it was the G.P. recommending it as she seemed stuck and is having to follow a protocol, not a neck or bone specialist whose advice I would trust a little more. But what real choice do I have? If I don't go, she will not refer me to anyone, and I cannot live like this.

My neck apparently looks twisted - the radiographer thinks as the muscles are tight, but she says there is nothing obviously wrong. She does another x-ray to check if the muscles are still showing as possibly tight or I was just leaning oddly, but apparently this one looks even worse. Then, as I said I was getting the x-ray as I have been feeling dizzy, had neck pain and was wanting a neurology appointment, she tells me that I would need another x-ray looking at the front of my neck. So I have three x-rays taken. Great.

As I leave she tells me the results will be with my G.P. within 7 days maximum. I query with her "will it not take 3 weeks I was told by the G.P?" and she insists no. So I go home to call the doctors surgery and book the next available G.P. appointment (this time with another locum) the earliest appointment is the 23rd March, 2 weeks away.

Each time we try and book an appointment with the GP it is taking ages- the earliest I can book is often 3 weeks away (unless they have just had a cancellation, or they have seemingly added a locum) and I have been told I need to book these routine appointments and not the emergency ones.

What else do I do? Dave says I should go to A&E, but I feel that is for accidents and emergencies- of which this is neither, and the NHS seem to be having a advertising spree saying it must only be used for this purpose, and you need to see your G.P for all else. Plus I don't want to think I am in an 'emergency' situation- and if I go there I will most likely have less of a say than I would if it was a routine appointment? I also know others are saying the NHS is slow, so accept this is just how things are.

15th March. I ask for support and so post this on a healing group on Facebook.

> *"I have suffered from mild balance issues for years, but damaged my neck (looking up when painting walls) in November and been getting a variety of pains from it since then.*
> *It has also increased the vertigo, tingling etc. so some days I barely want to move off the sofa. I have gone out when I felt bad, and fallen off a stool. I am now getting anxious with everything out of my comfort zone and every wobble is magnified.*
> *Various healing things have helped, but I cannot keep doing them too often (as cannot work, and Dave is having to look after me and house) I am slowly getting checks with GP (still waiting for neck referral, but heart, blood and ENT all ok)*
> *But please could you send any healing, strength, and calm & peaceful thoughts, as I am really not coping this week and now getting concerned there is something serious..."*

And this on a health support group as I was trying to follow a detoxing protocol:

> *"Hello. What do you do when you are totally fed up?*
> *Last year I pulled my neck and started sharp neck pains off, but it progressed to vertigo, unreality, tingling areas, weak legs, blurry eyes, no balance, a pounding head/neck ache if i turn wrong, and then anxiety when alone (plus with each period it has made the pounding head/neck really bad).*
> *It went off a bit when I stopped taking a B12 vitamin, but I have not felt fully ok since November. Tbh I am now scared that there is something really wrong - how do I know I don't have a brain tumour or something and I am putting it down to detox? I don't even eat that badly or drink alcohol... although I know my teens were toxic (physically plus*

*emotionally) - and this was when these symptoms started,
but MUCH milder. I know I have had them on and off ever
since -when I am down- for years, & have CFS, anxiety and
aches for years.*

*I gave up on Drs years ago (after they dosed me on years of
antibiotics) and have had natural therapies for years- and
had some tingling issues about 15 years ago, bad eyes,
unreality several times etc that did all clear up after a few
weeks ...*

*But now it's all of them together...and for months...
and I am really starting to not cope- I cannot even clean my
house, cook properly (if i do it all gets worse) and my poor
husband is having to look after me, cook dinner, sort the
house ... (the kids aren't doing anything I might ☹)*

*Do I assume that 'if' it was a brain tumour or anything I
wouldn't have had these things for years first?? I have had
basic tests from Dr, heart tests, blood tests, been to ENT, had
X-ray (which the radiographer said showed a twisted spine-
still waiting for full results) and supposed to be referred to
neuro/osteo consultant soon ... but I don't feel 'me'. ☹
Any thoughts appreciated x"*

Once again have a severe headache all over the back, front and top
of my head that seems to be hormonal as it arrives and goes with
my period. Most nights I am waking with a dull ache where I need
to move my head to release the pain. It seems if I sleep wrong and
bend my neck I wake up in agony, or with tingling in my head. And
the back of my head just feels it pounds at times. I am also still
getting an increase of the strange sensation when my head hurts
and the dizziness gets worse when I strain, cough or sneeze etc.

I decide to have a couple of craniosacral sessions, the therapist says
I am 'red lining' and need to take it easy. The headache seems to
get better afterwards and I even feel a bit less dizzy for a few days
each time. It seems to be similar when I have Bowen treatment, I

feel better after and it helps for a few days. But I cannot constantly have treatments, and it feels I need something every day.

I'm sitting at a friend's house with just a couple of other friends there and I just feel spaced out, I can't seem to follow the conversation and the lights are dim and it's annoying my eyes. I just feel I am having to be so careful all the time, just walking around someone else's house is like walking through the china department in a shop carrying loads of large bags sticking out everywhere. It's exhausting. No wonder I cannot concentrate.

This time Dave is playing a gig a thirty minute or so drive away, and it's a late finish. And guess who doesn't drink - so as normal I get the job of driving home. I'm on the A3 and I've decided that this is enough. I cannot do this anymore. The dizziness had been ok when I was in the car previously, like it somehow disappeared as the car was already moving differently to me. But if it's this late (1.30am) and I'm tired from now I am now refusing to drive. The road is too hard to concentrate on, there are no street lights so it's dark, pitch black, hardly any other cars are going the same direction where you can see and follow their tail lights, just cat's eye's lighting up in a few places... it feels I can't see anything, headlights come from the other direction and blind me ... I want to cry. Silent tears fall down my face as I mouth to ask the Angels to get us home safely. A car overtakes us and then stays at a distance I can follow which makes it easier. We get safely home and I leave Dave to unload the car as I go straight to bed letting the rest of the tears out.

Chapter 3 - What's wrong with me?

Finally we get to the next G.P. appointment on 23rd March and see another locum doctor. This time I take along a print out of all my current symptoms and concerns:

Loss of balance- feel I am on a boat. Hit objects as I walk past, or think I will.

Legs feel wobbly and weak.

Hurts when I turn round too fast/far (parking car is hard) then get dizzy

Occasional tingling/numbness in neck and head. (Like I've been laying on something hard)

Tightness on top of head, or back of head (between ear line – either above or behind)

Squinting to focus straight.

Back of head and neck (atlas joint?) pounds at times.

Definitely worse hormonally (started during a period and bad with each since- can feel around eyes too)

Head pains seems worse if I sleep wrong (if laying on my front with pillow, or tip neck up and back)

Both headache and unbalance worse when I cough, sneeze or strain. (If I put my head against the wall it seems ok!)

Occasional headache on front top of head.

Started neck pain when painting ceiling, but vertigo started getting bad a month or so after this.

Occasionally- Struggle to balance self with eyes- walking seems jolted and makes me feel unbalanced.

Clumsy!

Can I rule out?
Brain tumour or problem?
MS?

Chari malformation? neck pain, balance problems, muscle weakness, numbness or other abnormal feelings in the arms or legs, dizziness, vision problems, difficulty swallowing, ringing or buzzing in the ears, hearing loss, vomiting, insomnia, depression, or headache made worse by coughing or straining. Hand coordination and fine motor skills may be affected
Dyspraxia? (I have most of the symptoms!) Can I get tested? Irlen Syndrome? Some eye symptoms. Physical problems- Headaches & Migraines. Dizziness. Frowning. Mood swings in certain environments. Nausea. Sore, dry, red or watery eyes. Squinting Strain and fatigue. Stress from computers, reading and lighting. Tiredness. Stress. Panic. A feeling of disorientation. Restlessness.

As it's a different doctor again she does the hand eye coordination tests from my nose to her finger. Once again she again dismisses the chance it could be a brain tumour or Chairi as very unlikely, but this time says yes she will refer me to a neurologist and keeps the information I printed out.

The information I had printed was the only options I could see that possibly fitted my symptoms from Google. I had searched and searched various phrases over several days in desperation to find an answer and whilst it seems unlikely Chari malformation seems most relevant (albeit terrifying) for symptoms such as feeling worse when I cough or sneeze, and pains at the back of the head. Although I don't really want to read much too much more about it, the 'cure' is major brain surgery. I hope maybe an Irlen test and a pair of coloured contact lenses will stop this...

In the meantime I have a few more physiotherapy appointments - neither of the two therapists I've seen seem to think the dizziness could be related to the neck pain, and keep insisting that the neck exercises I have been given 'will' be helping. Even though I am telling them that when I do the exercises I seem to get more neck pain and headaches than if I don't do any. If I do the exercises before bed I wake more with violent headaches, if I do them by day I am dizzier directly after. I feel like I am going round in circles, or insane … the doctors and physiotherapists are telling me I am ok and basically implying 'it's all in my head'… when I feel awful and scared. Am I just sending myself slowly mad as I cannot focus on anything else? Is it really all just stress?

At various times during the above few months I have been increasingly and consistently seeing signs that lead me to various information on Angels. I admit I have had a deck of 'Healing with the Angel's' oracle cards for several years and many a time in the past they have helped me (e.g. when my Grandad died I got the same 'Support' card for five days in a row - chosen randomly from a muddled and unmarked pack of 44) and yet more and more things keep showing themselves to me that I should ask the Angels for guidance and support. So I am now daily asking Angels to help me, heal me, protect me, and to give me signs on what I should do. It seems most times I look at my phone I get a reversed or repeat number such as 12.21 or 19.19 and I also seem to see the 'Angel numbers' 11.11 (or 13.11 or 23.11) each day on the clock, as well as various other 111's. It might seem like nothing or just coincidence to others, but it feels I am being supported and helped.

25th March. I go to one more gig, this one is only a ten minute drive from home and it's not so late finishing, yet coming back in the dark after an evening of loud music and I feel the road is 'coming at me' and almost blurring as if I am looking at the side of a road when a passenger in a car driving at 70mph. I feel like I am driving at 60mph when I am doing 25 (and it's a 40mph road!) It's awful and scaring me badly. The road is lit, the road is straight and I know the road and where I am going, but I am physically feeling sick from how I feel and the lack of control. That's it - I am not driving home after a gig anymore. Dave will either have to agree to not drink or I just won't go.

I feel like I am giving in ... what is happening to me? I cannot now do what I always have. I feel old and useless. But this isn't just dizziness, it's far more severe, this is total physical exhaustion and I feel my body is no longer working right. Driving is a basic daily thing I have done for 24 years... but I just cannot do it anymore, and I don't know why. I'm failing big time.

I realise that I have written down that in March I have been dizzy every single day, had some kind of bad or constant head or neck pain every day plus 3 days of severe migraine like headaches where I basically can barely move from my bed to the sofa. Of which seem to be hormonal and related to my periods - am I getting bad hormonal migraines as I am getting older? I know that can happen to some people and my Mum and sister both are prone to migraines.

But the pain is insane. I have to follow a routine to even sit down - first I have to look down at the floor, then sit slowly and then gradually lift my head up. I am taking paracetamol (despite them making me feel nauseous and giving me belly pain), using the ibuprofen gel on my neck and still I feel I am all but twitching from the pain. We even call 111 - the NHS helpline - and get told to continue with the painkillers as they cannot see it's a serious problem. For a few days at a time I feel especially horrendous. I cannot even get in the shower- and this is from someone who never misses a shower to wash her hair each morning. What's wrong with me?

29th March. I did have another G.P. appointment booked, but I cancel it as the symptoms are no more horrendous than they were last week, and the last doctor said she was referring me to a neurologist, so what benefit would there be seeing someone else too? Plus the staff all ask you to cancel appointments if you can as they are needed by others. Yes if it takes 3-5 weeks to book to see someone I agree!

31st March. Text to Dave (He is out at a gig that I felt too ill to go to and texts to see how I am.)

> *"I am barely able to move as my head feels like its splitting open - even when I am still (and yes I have taken pain killers) And it's hard to communicate when you are in pain and the words aren't easy to even speak, or think ☹ "*

5th April. I ask on another health group for advice.

> *"Can I have your thoughts please to see if you think I am doing the right thing??*
> *I think I damaged my neck painting in November, (got sharp pains just after), started changing my diet a little in December and adding (too many?) supplements, In January I started having both 'on a boat/drunk' feelings and increasing neck and head pains. Headache has been getting worse with each period (I also get hormonal issues, but never had headaches before, much less with period) this month (last week) it was like a nail being hammered in for 4 days - horrendous! Far worse than any labour!! ☹*
> *But over the last few days although I have felt awful with my head, I felt I wasn't constantly 'on the boat' (though still had dizziness when coughing or got up too quick- seemingly more related to the neck?) and like the dizziness was getting better.*
> *But again today I feel the boat is back ☹*

*Could supplements be causing the drunken feelings, or do
you think they would have contributed to my neck and head
pain? And is there any logical way it would cause the
hormonal headache?
I have spent 3 months basically unable to go out alone, and
have unreality panics if i do...."*

6th April- It's my birthday! Mum comes over to try and help me do
some jobs in the garden I want to do but have not been able to
manage. I attempt to plant a few seedlings in pots outside and yet I
can barely bend down, get dizzy each time I turn, wobble as I lean
or move. I can't carry anything - even carrying a fairly light pot
makes my head pound so much it feels it's going to burst, and I'm
exhausted. It's crap. There is something really wrong and I am
afraid. Terrified for the future, or this being my new future. Is this
going to be my last birthday?

Although I have finally got my neurologist appointment on the NHS
through... for 23rd May, hardly quick! I guess we are constantly told
the NHS is underfunded and therefore very slow and over run and I
will have to wait.

So as basically everyone has said (when I think they have exhausted
their ideas) I should rest... but I have barely moved of the sofa for a
month, resting my neck is clearly not helping the pain, and I am able
to do less and less by the day. What's wrong with me???

On 10th April, I really want to go to a Creative Day that was being held locally by Hollie Holden. I know I need to work out how to mix my need for creativity with being a mum of four, and one with low energy at that, and her 'Notes on Living and Loving' often resonate with me. I had contacted them a week or so before to let me know if there were spaces and if I could pay cash on the day if I felt well enough to go as I was having severe dizziness problems. They did, so I trust that it is right for me to go and I end up driving there one Sunday morning somewhat feeling I need to go, but also that I am freaking out. I am so confused, spaced out and not knowing what is going on. I have to keep on sunglasses while driving as they seem to help my vision, stop the road moving too quickly at me and keep me in control of what I'm feeling. At the event (which was small group where you all bring food to share) I feel I have to move slowly and deliberately and almost that I need to hold on to walls. I can't turn properly and feel really slow. It seems like a duel reality where I was happy and calm and enjoying the day on one hand and yet in a total panic and exhausted on another.

At one point Hollie explained a little bit about Rudolf Steiner's belief that at age 42 we have a spiritual birth. That at this time, the soul has the opportunity to a higher state of consciousness called Spirit Self. She says that many people she knows had something significant (illness, divorce, change of career) happen to them at this age, my age. Yes, something feels significant about this year, I don't know what but I know I've never felt this so clearly before. Towards the end of the day we also find various pictures and quotes to cover a journal with. Some quotes I stuck on my book cover, although I didn't really understand why I wanted to keep them, but I did. The event feels honest and real and I really do feel it has helped me, although by the time I get home I am shattered.

Just before we left one of the other participants, Tina, announces that she has been starting to work with Angel cards and messages and with the friends and family she had helped so far they had found the messages helpful. She offered to give those of us there a free reading over the following few weeks if we wanted it. I take her details.

At this point I have decided I'm not driving anymore - at all. I feel awful. I cannot turn. Everything seems so hard to do. The road is coming at me and I don't feel safe anymore. Not to mention that my head aches most nights, either the front area over my eyes or the back area, so badly it constantly wakes me up. I have sharp pains up my neck and into my head. I'm not able to walk anywhere straight and feel I am bumping into people or walls all the time. My anxiety is through the roof - I feel I am going mad. Or dying.

Chapter 4 - The Battle in my Head

12th April. Written in journal. Inspired after creative day to write my emotions down.

Vertigo

It doesn't even sum it up
Even the name is not right
I'm not even spinning
I just feel like I am drunk
On a boat, had a shock
Or woken unexpectedly from a sleep
I just cannot walk straight
Keep hitting the wall
Veering from side to side
Unable to balance.
Then my legs feel weak
A rush of adrenaline
To stop you falling
But you weren't going to fall
... just wobble
Driving a car feels so hard
You 'really' have to focus
As everything feels it is coming at you
... too fast
You feel you are losing your balance
Just looking at the road
Even though you are sitting down!
Shopping is torture
You think everyone will assume
That you are drunk
When you hit a wall
Or are unable to move out the way
Bump into someone.

And the lights
Oh hell!
They seem to pulse into your soul
Like waves in the sea
Draining all your power
Until you collapse from exhaustion
Crying at home
Again.
A simple task is a marathon
Using all your resources
Your willpower and strength
You want to cook the dinner
Do some gardening
Yet you cannot keep turning around
Even twice is enough
For the feeling of 'oh hell
-this is like torture'
I feel like I am dying
How do I know that I'm not?
Or is this just healing me and making me rest?
As sitting down and not
Looking at a screen
I feel normal
For a while
I am free.
But I don't have a servant
To do all my chores
I have to rest
To accept I am drunk
For a girl that doesn't drink
As long ago it stopped being fun
Ask the angels to heal me
To guide me
Accept its part of the plan
Soak in the sun's rays
And know I'll do what I can

13th April

What is upsetting me?

I am exhausted, shattered, emotionally and physically fatigued
I feel I am shaking on the inside from a deep fear
I don't even understand

My soul is crying, my soul is dying
And I have no idea how to get it back

I feel I need to go away to a secluded warm beach
And just stare into the waves
Throw stones in the sea

Let my tears merge with the water until I can cry no longer
My soul has been rocked calm by the movement

Then at night I can just look at the stars
Until I am connected to the universe
Healed in the universal power

Retreat is not defeat

Retreat is not defeat
I chose this quotation
Even then I didn't fully understand
That it's not just time to slow
But now is the time to heal

Retreat into my past
Go back to the whole me
The last time I remember being free
Unworried by life, unconcerned about death
Just living in the moment and happy

It's so far back in time, there's just a hint left
Of the last time I was truly ME
But now my head has told me to stop
Physically made me sit
Let go of the should's, the guilt and belief's

Just stop
And let go
Accept that's all over
Now it's time to find me again
To heal that inner child

To love that teen
To hold her strong
Help let out her fears instead of silence
It's all so much worse bottled inside
They eat you alive

So I sit, and I write
And I draw, and I cry
And listen to that teen, who died inside
Help her heal
Heal from the emotional scars

Let her reconnect to the strength that's hers
The love she was born with
The strength in her heart
The trust the world is there for her
If she just asks inside

So while I'm retreating
Just allow me to be
I know I am healing
Not defeated
But allowing me to be me.

The battle in my head

It's a daily fight
The battle in my head
Do I listen to the fears & the dramatic stories?
And can I control them?

But they will not be held back
Supressed they just breed more
Until my whole day is one black hell
Of fear, of pain, of tears

And I long for sleep to release me
To be at peace, in that between place
Of life and death
The very two things I fear

And if I have the strength- I can allow it
Feel the weakness, the out of control-ness
The pain, the fears, the anger, the frustration
And … just let them be

If I die…it's got to be better than this
So death can be accepted. And I trust.
Trust that Grace will provide for me
That I am safe, a wreck- but ashore

And sometimes it can go.
Burnt away in the flames of trust
Released to the world for it to take away
To set me free

Chapter 5 - Verge of a Breakdown

14th April. Text to Dave.

> *"I feel I am SO on the verge of a breakdown - so fucking close - as everything is raw!!"*

In desperation I try a chiropractor as it's one of the only treatments I have never tried, and I don't think anything I have ever tried before will work. If it's my neck that's causing these problems from a trapped nerve or something then he should know. I get Dave to take me to the appointment and the chiropractor clicks and cracks my neck, each time asking me does it feel better, but I still feel dizzy and unbalanced. Then when I say how anxious I feel he kindly suggests I should go jogging or do some decent exercise to calm me down! I try to explain that this would do the opposite to me for various reasons, but he just continues to tell me the times that strenuous exercise helped him and how it brings oxygen to the organs. When I continue to tell him this won't work for me (especially at the moment) and my reasons why - I just get mocked. Dave picks me up and I get in the car and cry. I feel humiliated and misunderstood and unless he doesn't know anything - it isn't my neck...

The next day - after listening to me sobbing for much of it- Dave calls my Mum and asks if she and my Dad would be able to help him pay to see a doctor privately. That we need to do something and the NHS just isn't doing anything fast enough. We have listened over the past few months what happened with my uncle going through the slow NHS system and eventually diagnosed with cancer after several weeks of nothing happening and lost appointments. We need to chase this up. Mum agrees and speaks to a consultant doctor friend of theirs, who after listening to what happened and the ENT doctor saying it was likely my neck gives us the details of a rheumatologist he works with as it seems the best choice for now - and the rheumatologist could then refer me if need be. So we book an appointment for early the following week.

I have a ticket booked to see Muse at the O2 on Friday 15th April, all week I don't think I will be able to go - the last thing I want is to go out and have a panic attack from feeling so bad and freaking out, ruin it for my kids that are going too. But I also really don't want to miss it either (listening to Muse live, with all the stadium singing along is just the best) and know I will be very annoyed with myself if I don't get there. In the end (on the Friday) I decide I am going - I take some Homeopathic Gelsenium for the anxiety, ask the Angels (a lot!) to support me and trust I will be ok … Somehow I manage to accept the 'drunkenness', pretend I am drunk and get on with it.

Walking in the tube stations where there are lots of people coming the other way is just awful... it is like my head is going insane and I cannot focus properly and everything is just bouncing along too fast in the opposite direction. My vision on 'jumping camera mode' again. I just continue to focus on the back of my eldest son who is walking in front of me to clear me a pathway, move my legs and keep trusting. Walking around the stadium is ridiculous, as it's a curve, a large curve but certainly not in a straight line. I just feel so drunk. Stupid and drunk. If someone had said they had spiked my drink or I had just drunk neat vodka I would have believed them.

Then we are on the highest tier of the stadium! Admittedly only a few row back, but the top level. I can only walk up to my seat holding on to the handrails with both hands, then holding on the backs of the chairs as I walk along the row to get to my chair. Terrified that I will fall over and crash down on the steep rows of seating beneath us as my balance is so bad. People kindly end up holding their hands out to me so I can move along the row as I said I was so scared and had a dizziness problem at the moment!

I post to Facebook.

> *"Fuck it's high here! Not good with dizziness!!! I want a seatbelt..."*

Text to Dave.

> *"Got here ok. Escalators don't help, nor does being super high up!! I look seriously drunk and feel my legs have gone, but all good!"*

Then the music starts. It chills me. Several times I just sit and shut my eyes, tears rolling down my cheeks, listening to the music, the lyrics, and the whole stadium singing along - really feeling inside me the power of the experience. The power of unity. The power of trust.

19th April. Back to reality and the private doctor's appointment. I am crying in the car going there, I need Dave to help me out the car and hold me to walk into the hospital as I am so wobbly. I walk in the room with the list I gave the last G.P, but in less than a month I had added the following in a different coloured text to that original list:

When bad - if I go to sit down I have to look down at floor, sit, then gradually look up. If I don't I have severe waves of pain, and dizzy after. I feel my eyes flicker?

Hormonal headache- such a severe pain that I feel I am jolting/twitching when I move my neck, get up etc

Lifting my head when laying on my front is agony! Severe pains, both sharp and ache all around atlas. Feel dizzy. Eyes feel odd and want to just move back and put head on floor and cry.

My neck cracks/grates when I turn it now- been told arthritis by physio- but didn't have it before December.

It is now totally taking over my life- I cannot go out alone, panic when I do if get dizzy. Headaches starting in night (3am >) I can't sleep. Driving at night harder- car/street lights too bright, road feels it's 'coming at me'. Don't feel my legs are connected to brain.
Know I am totally stressed – both physically and mentally. Tired. Tearful. Depressed. Exhausted.

The worse headaches start with period- gradually increasing in pain. Most of the night I could not get comfy, had to sit up on pillows. Couldn't get to sleep until 1ish. Woke at 4 with severe pain that lasted until 8-9. Went back to sleep soundly until 10-11. When got up the pain got better. Almost felt ok at times. (but hurt if got up and went to loo etc)
Took paracetamol and used ibuprofen gel which numbed some of the pain but I could still feel it. (and I DON'T take pain killers. Taking 2 tablets gave me nausea, even when taken with food!)

Headache had started to go away, but came back as I had a cold! Couldn't blow my nose as head felt it would explode. Sitting on sofa barely able to move and just crying from pain. Pains with both period and cold mainly in back -right of atlas, transferring to back of right eye, and sometimes top of head. Huge waves of pain in neck/back of head whenever I moved – so that I felt I was twitching with pain.

Now-
Atlas area hurts, and sometimes pounds, when I move head wrong- especially if turn to look slightly behind me to right, and I also get dizzy at same time. Often have muscles in knots in neck. Am limited in so much ☹

Want to know I am not causing any damage when I turn etc as it feels something is very wrong to hurt this much.

Like the first GP, after asking the basics on what is wrong, he asks me to do the simple neurological tests. I can still touch my finger to my nose and his moving finger alright and the ear balance tests are ok, but I still cannot walk in a straight line nor put my feet touching in front of each other. The exact same 'drink drive' test I did three months before. I joke that I didn't fall over and I was better than I was in January, or I felt I was. But I was still awful and I couldn't touch one heel to toe.

Almost as soon as I do this he strongly recommends I should get an MRI to check for a rare condition. I know he says some possible problem in the brain, but I didn't take in what, but one that presents itself as being 'drunk' when you are not actually drunk, which I am, and so I need to have an MRI to rule it out.

He sits us down, listens to a few of the symptoms written on my list and says he will give me the preliminary diagnosis of Occipital Neuralgia - but clearly states that I don't really fit all the symptoms of it and it doesn't fit all of mine. He says if I was older or had family history he would also consider a mini stroke!! He gives me the advice for what to do if it is Occipital Neuralgia so I don't have to pay for a follow up appointment if the MRI is ok, but we agree I 'need' to get an MRI as soon as possible (which my parents had already agreed they would pay for). It is still another 5 weeks before the appointment date to see the neurologist on the NHS and that wasn't even a possible scan date. A scan would most likely take even longer … and I neither he nor I feel I should wait.

I walk out of the doorway from the consulting room and almost into the corridor wall as I just continue going round the corner…

I call Mum to confirm the cost of the MRI he suggested (I have been advised to have both my head and neck scanned) and book it for the soonest date they can make, a few days away.

19/4/16. Written in Journal:

> "Got to see rheumatologist today. Possibly have occipital neuralgia- well as long as the MRI does not show up anything bad.
> Asking angels to help me to heal, the scan be ok & be calm. But I feel like I'm going round in circles, who to ask what, what should I check, who do I see… do I take medicines, injections etc or just let go and trust?
> What can I do to stop me thinking I am a freak?"

Chapter 6 - My Bloody Brain Tumour

Three days later I am back to get my MRI, it feels like a drunken dream. Everything is so hard to do and focus on as it feels it's constantly moving - wrongly. I lie down on the scanner and tell the nurse I am shutting my eyes as I don't want to look when I am inside the scanner and feel shut in, but also that I am still then - when my eyes are shut I finally stop spinning. Once again I ask the Angels to protect me and I trust them. For an hour I lie there listening to my meditation CD playing through the scanner and trusting that I need this done and trying to keep calm. The machine clunks, clicks and whirls around, I can feel myself moving in it. But I trust. They stop it briefly and say they need to give me the contrast dye injection that they said before was a possibility, and while my normal self would have totally refused it, I just say ok. Somehow I know I need it.

I go home, have some lunch and sit down, and my mobile phone rings... it's the consultant. He tells me he needs to discuss the MRI results with me and can I get back up to the hospital that afternoon...

As I sit down at the consultant's desk - he flicks through these pictures on his screen. Even I can see I have a brain tumour. A 3cm white blob on my scan - quite obviously not belonging there.

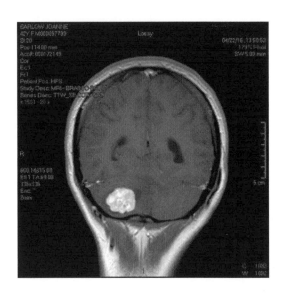

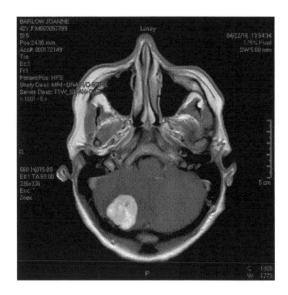

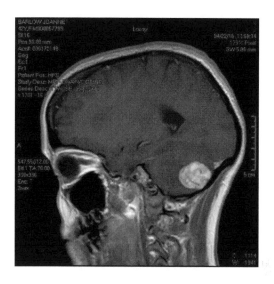

The consultant tells us the neuroradiologist who did the scan said he was 99% sure it was a hemangioblastoma (or haemangioblastoma) as they look different to most tumours - a benign blood vessel tumour, but one that needs removing ASAP. They would operate and remove it and it is quite a straightforward operation now. I would need referring back to the NHS and would be seen by a neurosurgeon within 2 weeks (as it is a tumour- which technically could be cancerous). Shaking, I ask him how do they get at it and do they shave my hair off, and he says they would just cut the back part of my hair and access the bottom part of the skull. That feels a bit better than the top of my head. I don't know why.

I ask why they would operate ASAP and when would it be, but he says "I am sorry I am not a neurologist and don't know the exact details or the normal procedure - only what the neuroradiologist has told me when he gave me the scan report. But do go to St George's A&E if you have further issues or deterioration or the pain gets worse. St George's Hospital have by far the best neurosurgery department in the area." I actually felt sorry for him as he told me - he looked upset.

We leave his office, with a letter for my G.P. to refer me back to the NHS. I am in shock. Tears streaming from my eyes. Somehow everything is in slow motion too and unreal - like it's some kind of sick joke someone is playing on me.

We get in the car and Dave drives me back down the A3. As its late Friday afternoon I call the doctors surgery to see if they are still open to hand in my referral letter - yes they are there for another hour. My cousin calls me on my mobile about an issue she is having and wanted my advice, and I blankly tell her my news. She sounds shocked too, and I think we both just said 'oh my god' and 'fuck' a lot.

Dave and I go straight to the G.P. surgery with the referral letter to get seen by a neurosurgeon at St George's ASAP. It feels like my life, the chance of keeping my life, is in this letter.

We walk into the G.P. surgery. The young lad behind the reception desk is laughing with someone out the back, he sees my note to the Dr and shuts up, looking embarrassed. Scans the letters and says he will pass it on to the doctors for referral now.

I get home and go straight up to bed... I can't talk to anyone. I can't talk to the kids. I can't phone my Mum and tell her it was all ok... I just cry into this empty void...

Half an hour or so later Dr Strickland, one of the partner doctors at the G.P. surgery, calls up and tells me he has just received my letter. He tells me he will forward it along with his covering letter, to St George's Hospital at 8am on Monday morning. If there is anything they can do, please contact him. I know I cannot say much, I can't even think properly, but I say something about "It was failing the same 'drink drive walking test' that I did with your G.P. in January that the private Doctor said I needed a MRI. I couldn't do either of them, although this time I think I did it better." But he just went quiet and muttered something about getting the referral done.

Dave eventually tells my parents and the older kids. I think they are in shock too. But I can't listen, I can't talk to them, I can't even admit it to myself yet. And I really can't tell my 'baby' (even though he is 9 ½ years old, but the other three are 6-12 years older than him, so he is my baby) that it's a brain tumour in case he has heard something bad about them - as after all you only hear about people dying of cancerous brain tumours, within months. So Dave and then I tell him I have a lump in my neck that needs an operation to remove it. Maybe that thought suits me too?

22.4.16. Journal entry.

> "So I have MRI done and feel dizzy but ok, stayed calm having it done by listening to Abraham meditation CD. Even got injected with dye and felt it was ok to have it. Go home. Got call 1 hour later saying I was to come back and discuss. Shit. Feel sick. Barely able to walk. Feel lightheaded. Panicky. Shaky. Terrified.
> Thinking I either have a brain tumour and I'm dying, or I have severe MS (and why I'm so dizzy). Cannot stop crying.
>
> Sitting in car I have a clear vision of walking up my front pathway to my house as a kid with my Nan following me, admiring my red curls, saying "I hope you never have a brain tumour and they need to cut them curls off" ...oh fuck.
>
> Get there, need loo. Go into consultant's room and he shows me I have a cyst type structure in my brain. A fucking tumour. A large white lump that shouldn't be there. Cannot stop crying even more. Scared I will die. Scared of the fact I have to see Doctors, hospitals and trust them...oh hell!
>
> Is this my life over? My kids, I don't want to hurt my kids.

Got told it's in cerebellum and they want to operate ASAP and Dr's see this type of tumour (the neuroradiologist is 99% sure it's this type) as a 'good one to remove'. I ask "So is it better than 'you have 3 months to live'?" and get told "No it's not like that at all, it can be removed by surgery and no it cannot suddenly go (burst)". Which calms me a little- I have time to think. But oh- I am ill. Really have something up. I wasn't just imagining it, I am sick. I have a tumour affecting my balance.

I cannot stop shaking, sobbing and am so scared. I need a brain op!!!! Yes it's not my 'thinking brain' and for that I am relieved, but it's an operation. On my brain. I'm scared. It feels like some of the world has stopped. How do I enjoy anything ever again? I want it out and gone ...now! I want to be normal again.

And why didn't I see before? Why didn't I realise? Why didn't the G.P. in January? Would it have made it better? Easier to operate on? Am I going to make it through the operation? What if I don't? What will happen to the kids? Do I write them a goodbye note? What will happen with my next period- will I have a severe headache again? And is this now dangerous? And I can't have the op during my period or full moon as I am sure I will bleed more and that's not good. Oh fuck. I want someone to look after me. Tell me what to do (and not) ...but I am the one who knows this stuff (not Dave or family)...so it's all down to me... and... I am terrified.

How do I want to be buried? But I don't want to die. I have my kids I want to see be adults. Even my 'baby'. I cannot leave him- I just cannot."

I'm numb. I can barely walk. I can barely move. I feel so sick I cannot eat. I now feel that 'I know what is causing all my problems - a fucking brain tumour' so I cannot manage to even attempt to try and hold it together anymore. I can't ignore my dizziness or my drunkenness, I can't ignore my headache, my neck pain, the pounding, the fact I cannot turn. It's not going to go away. I don't need to try and pretend everything is all ok anymore. It's not. It wasn't just an unexplained cause, a minor cause, a trapped nerve or something I had been eating or doing. IT'S A FUCKING BRAIN TUMOUR!!! I just cry and cry until I feel I have run out of tears. Constantly shaking inside. I need Dave to hold me, someone to help me. My skull needs to be opened. I'm terrified. Totally fucking terrified.

Chapter 7 - Doing My Head In

I somehow manage to get myself dressed, albeit I cannot manage a shower, especially not alone, as I can just about tie my hair up and wash; and get downstairs each day and just sit and watch TV. I can't do much else and I need something to take my mind off this. Problem being I don't really watch or like TV. I start with animal documentaries, but soon I am fed up of watching one animal be killed by another. Why does something always have to die? The natural world shows just make me disgusted with how much humans abuse our planet, and how much we disrespect ancient cultures who make far more sense to me than the idiots running much of the world now. I cannot watch the shows on travel or having a 'dream build' - bloody snooty people who have a million pounds to spend but don't appreciate it and get cross because something is slightly the wrong shade of brown! In the end I start to watch the 'Big Bang Theory' series, back to back, for what feels like days at a times with only the peace of sleep in between. Sometimes I cannot manage to watch it, the screen seems to move around too much. And then I cannot watch as Amy is cutting up a brain or two and finding tumours! But I listen- or try and just read the subtitles - it helps me switch off and takes my mind off of panicking.

23rd April. Text to Dave -he has gone to a gig that he had booked saying it would help him to be normal still.

> *"Gone to bed. Am ok. But tired and stressed with what will happen, and all the 'what if's' and so fed up with feeling fucking drunk.*
> *And I need a hug- for a few hours!* ♥ ♥ ♥ *"*

24/4/2016. Journal Entry:

> "Ok. So I have been told I have a cerebellar brain tumour!!! A big white lump that shouldn't be there on the screen with fluid all around it. It needs operating on to remove it ASAP. Bolloxs.
>
> Have ordered frankincense oil and asked the Angels. Roan has started taking the energy away- A pure healing love of serenity (he said he could feel cold when he started – and then it went)
>
> I feel it's going... I think working through all my past emotions has made it worse and gave me the symptoms. All those things that have 'done my head in'. The swelling and fluid is my body trying to heal it- taking the lump of fear away.
>
> I even had a dream a few nights ago...of doing a large hard poo standing up in front of my family! But I just put my hand down and got rid of it! Saying the crap is going, the past stuff is going. I felt the feeling of huge relief and a weight gone. Soothing once it had gone. I was free and able to be me. The shit was out.
>
> So I am asking my tumour what it needs to tell me and listening...."

(I use a technique I have used before where I write questions to my higher-self using my right hand, and reply back using my left hand)

> "Dear cerebellar tumour. Please tell me what I need to do to get rid of you and get my balance back?"
>
> "Listen to Grace, not to your fears. I am a lump of all your pain, hurt, fears, lack of self-worth, anger, hate, sadness, pity and not doing what you are truly capable of.

I've been here years. Since you gave up on yourself as a teen. You lost your dreams, passion, your Faith in Grace, knowing that you are always safe and protected.
I hurt as you were acknowledging them, but still not really listening and not understanding. But you do now x ❤ x
I can go now, but you have to be you. Powerful and strong. What you were made for.
Let go and trust"."

Occasionally when the weather is good I get outside and sit on my sunbed in the garden. I accept that I walk there looking and acting like I am drunk, falling over the stones and pathway, with my hands held out to balance myself. But then just sit and breathe in nature and the universe. My vision seems a little better as the longer distance seems to help me feel less like I am spinning, and the clouds move as you look at them anyway. At times I can lie back and sunbathe, looking at the sky and forget about it all for a few minutes. The sun seems to heal me.

But most of the time I feel so out of control, I can barely walk even to the loo and back and when I do I hit the walls in the hallway. I can't concentrate, I can't even speak straight and articulate my feelings properly. Yet I am supposed to continue and get on with things, when all the time I feel I am waiting for the executioner to arrive.

I'm numb. I still can't think straight. I want to look up possible alternatives and what my tumour actually is, what the cause is. Problem being I can barely look at a computer screen without getting travel sickness type nausea as I cannot see it properly. I struggle to type as my brain cannot work out which keys are which. I have to focus on every letter as I type and spell out each word in my head.

I ask on some energy healing Facebook groups for advice - and mainly get told to look at Cannabis oil and Frankincense. But my tumour isn't cancer, it's not even a 'normal' benign tumour from what I can gather. It's the blood vessels that are screwed up...can 'anything' help with that?

There is barely anything I can find online about Hemangioblastoma … and half of what I do find is aimed at Dr's or surgeons, and I don't want to read that. I'm not ready for it. It's too graphic.

I order some food grade frankincense oil. It is expensive but I want to try and see if it will help. If I can shrink it, even just a bit. I put a couple of drops on my tongue each day - its tastes of medicine and is disgusting, but I trust. I have to. I have no other option.

I look up brain tumours with my Louise Hay 'You can heal your life' book (so many times in the past this book has been accurate and helped me) and for the brain it says the 'probable cause' - 'Represents the computer, the switchboard' and the new thought pattern should be "I am the loving operator of my mind".

For brain tumours the cause being 'incorrect computerised beliefs. Stubborn. Refusing to change old patterns.' And the new thought pattern being "It is easy for me to reprogram the computer of my mind. All of life is change and my mind is ever new." I also see (and have known this from elsewhere) that blood and blood vessels represent the joy of life.

Eeek! That hurts. I know my thoughts can be rubbish. I know I am holding on to old beliefs. I know I am stubborn and refuse to change old patterns. It's what I have been working on these last few years-to get rid of my demons! And for sure my joy is stagnating... in one big lump that's literally doing my head in?!

Each night, I just cry and cry at Dave getting him to hold me. I need someone to protect me. Stop this horrid nightmare. It helps - just.

26th April - Tuesday afternoon. I am panicking and wanting to know what is happening with my 'ASAP operation' and when would I even see the consultant to ask the many questions and worries I have. Something is telling me I need to call St George's Hospital and find out. So while Dave has gone out briefly I manage to look up St George's neurosurgery department online and call them. They ask for my details and after a while the receptionist comes back and tells me I am not on the computer system, nor in the tray of paperwork they have received that day about to get on their computer system. So she tells me it is unlikely my G.P. has even sent them my details! This is like some sick joke the G.P surgery is playing - with my life. I am given her name and fax number (the NHS still fax?!) and told to call my G.P. surgery and get them to send the referral letter directly to her now.

So I call the surgery. The guy on the reception (possibly the same person I saw the previous Friday) listens and says he will re send the fax while I am on the phone, and then a minute or so later confirms it has been sent. So half an hour later I call St George's neurosurgery back and confirm with them they have received it - yes they have now got my referral details. Although the woman tells me I have now missed that days 'emergency cases meeting' and so my details won't now be seen until Thursday!

How could a doctor who promised me he would send this form off at 8am the day before have not checked it got there? I want to scream. How useless can the G.P. surgery actually be? They have failed me miserably so far this year and just done it again.

Chapter 8 - I Have to Trust

Online I find a brain tumour support group 'brainstrust' and they have a Facebook page. I search for Hemangioblastoma and find an old post from someone who had the same tumour removed also from her cerebellum just over a year before. She is ok. Alive and well. She tells me she has a numb head still and a few odd problems, but basically says she is fine and can now forget about it. I find out she also had her operation at St George's too and lives locally. The relief of hearing this is enormous! I cry out all my worries and concerns and she says the operation was quite severe as she was in special care for a few days or so but then home after a week and able to do normal things a few weeks later. I am terrified of being in special care for a week...I am a control freak and don't want to be 'out of it'. Fuck. I don't drink partly as I cannot stand the feeling, I don't take medicines well and always seem to get the side effects. How will I manage being in special care?

Oh, but she didn't get all her hair cut off!! They just shave the back area (near the neckline) where the cut will be, and it's under the rest of your hair so not like a bald patch really visible on the top of your head. It sounds pathetic to be worrying over hair compared with what they are going to do... but it feels like someone is saying they don't have to chop a limb off as well during the operation.

27th April. Just had this in my inbox- from Mike Dooley - Notes from the universe.

> "ZINGER ALERT:
>
> When life hurts, Jo. When it baffles and confuses. When it doesn't quite seem to work. These are just signs from Me, as

if I were tapping on your shoulder or whispering in your ear, trying to point out that something important, something really, really important, is being misunderstood.

This Note is just in case, one day, something doesn't make sense. You know, for a friend.

Warm hugs,
The Universe"

I just cry. Tears seem to be the only thing I can do well at the moment.

I send a text to Nicola (a friend who does Gaia healing work)

"I am struggling- feeling very panicky at times and really don't know what to do. Asking Angels and trusting and a bit of aconite (a homeopathic remedy) *gradually helps it go off. Scared shitless of surgery- on my fucking brain!! – Although hospitals and bleeps terrify me, so not sure what I can do?*

Must admit, if I can get over this, I can get over anything!!!! They have finally seen my scan etc at St George's. It's been a right fuck up since January on all counts- St George's said they will phone back between today and Friday with what's happening. But I am terrified as have not yet seen surgeon and have spent 5 days with no info and lots of 'what if's' ... am trying to be positive but tbh failing... but apparently that's normal!

All healing gratefully received ♥ *"*

Maybe if you don't hear or worry about ambulance and police sirens going past your house, you won't understand my fear on the hospital bleeps. I cannot listen to even TV programmes with these sounds on as I can feel the fear and anger rising in me. It's like something is crawling inside my body and I just start to freak...

I know many other people don't like hospitals, but when you also have a distrust of what many doctors and nurses believe in, as well as what they say and do. Don't tolerate drugs well. Don't like being out of control. Have a fear that they will do something I wouldn't agree with when I am in no fit state to give my opinion... plus feel an odd empathy for others who are ill -as though it's me that's in their boat. Maybe people will understand the panic the thought of even a night in hospital brings.

Yet I can't see a brain operation only being one night?! I know many people trust they are in 'good hands' when they go to hospital. I don't. It's like now I have to be extra alert and prepared for what is happening.

But I have to trust... I have no option but to let go. I can't do brain surgery on myself and I totally believe in healing. I believe in stories such as Anita Moorjani where she was in a coma from stage 4 lymphatic cancer and while in the coma also had a near death experience where she chose to come back to continue to live, and despite all the odds and the doctors saying her organs were shutting down - she healed.

All day I keep seeing what I now call Angel numbers: 11:11, 12:21, 13:31 etc. It seems like they are telling me it will be alright. Whatever happens.

I realised that where I asked for help, advice and healing on a Facebook energy medicine group, I have now got 100's of comments and replies- some technical, some I will look at more, some I instantly resonate with, some ideas I don't want to do...but lots of love and healing comments. Funny how people you don't know being kind seems to help. Or maybe it isn't - after all we are all human. And I truly believe in the power of group healing and intention. This is the sort of information I have been reading about for years...

And so I text back to Nicola later:

> *"Finally got the calmness and that whatever happens is for my healing (tho still 100% believe it can heal, or start to, before op - if that is my path)*
> *Especially as I have barely had any headache or sharp pains in a week, when before they were daily- or even constant for months!*
> *I need to keep feeling this- especially as Dave is unbelieving that healing can happen whether from self or others. And none of the (mainstream) medical stuff talks about alternatives – obviously!*
> *Also brought Frankincense oil- £80!! – from doTerra and been putting on both roof of mouth and base of skull xx*
> *The brainstrust help line say this type of tumour is truly benign- so not sure if it's like a cyst (the original Dr said that word) which isn't cancer or a 'not expected to spread' tumour. Deep down I feel it's as I really addressed my past, yes something has been there for years- from the causes that have hurt me - did my head in- and this made it worse...*
> *Something is changing, still dizzy, but no pain has got to be something?!*
> *Plus asked the Angels out loud a few times today, as well as the whispers, and the shivers in me after has been immense. And actually ate dinner and enjoyed it- first time in weeks* ☺
>
> *Am now going to trust it (and try not to focus on the wobbles and my negativity xx)"*

But at night... I just want to cry. Want Dave to rescue me somehow. Even his holding me feels it helps a little, although I somehow want him to hold my head and fix it too. Or tell me it was just a nightmare I am having and that I have now woken and everything is ok. I'm scared. I don't know what's happening - apart from I need an operation ASAP. Why is it so urgent? Apart from I feel crap. What is the risk?

28th April. Text from and to Nicola (after saying I am scared)

> (From Nicola: It's ok to allow that fear to come up, just acknowledge that it is there, thank it and tell it that's its ok.
> Say something like 'thank you fear, pass through me now and move on, as I don't need you right now'
> Breathe through it, feel it and gently let it go
> Recognise that you are (I am) not this fear (i.e. – don't identify with it) just acknowledge its energy passing through
> As for gratitude and 'I am's' I wouldn't even mention or refer to a tumour (as at the causal level it's already gone, right) in the physical it's in the process of leaving.
> So just say something like 'I am in perfect health and balance. I am fully aligned in perfect health and I thank you for this blessing of peace, health and harmony' or 'thank you universe (God, Source etc.) for my perfect expression of health in body, mind and spirit... (Be playful and creative as you make up ones you like and that you can relate to)
> Thank you for all the wisdom and blessings these experiences are bringing me, which are for my highest good...)

To Nicola:

> *"Thank you so much for your words, healing and asking others for me too* ❤ ❤ ❤ *but you know it's the first time I*

have ever felt truly cared for and loved unconditionally by others! (I need a brain tumour to do it!?) It's like its magnified all the love my family have times 1000 as most people don't even know me but still care

I had over 130 replies to a post on 'energy medicine exchange' and the power of that feels amazing xx and others have added me to their own group prayer lists etc...I am going to stay in those thoughts for a while ♥ "

Text to Alison

"I don't know if you will agree but I am still believing and asking for healing from others and angels etc- I know I had many times of terror and not been calm, but deep down feel that whatever happens it will make me stronger and believe in myself more. And I feel the worst of my panic fears are over...I now need to trust ♥ "

At times I can feel fully trusting and positive and then I can descend into total despair within a few minutes. It is another day and another mix of every emotion under the sun. Some at the same time! How is it possible to feel both extreme fear and joy at once? Not knowing is the hardest part as I am sure my imagination is worse than any reality. Dave calls up St George's neurosurgery and finds out that after the meeting I am scheduled as a priority case. I am in category 1 (out of 3 - category 1 being the most urgent) and they have discussed my case, but not yet sorted a date to see the consultant.

Knowing you are the most urgent of new cases due to have brain surgery at a top neurosurgery hospital is terrifying, although I actually laugh when I realise! How things can change in a few weeks and how grateful we paid for a private MRI.

I again ask my body to talk to me - again by writing to myself using both hands.

29/4/2016. Journal Entry:

"Ok tumour, do I need to know anything more?"

"That I am glad you listened. I know you have really heard me. You still have to keep implementing it, to make sure you are true to you. It doesn't matter if people take it the wrong way if said and meant with LOVE.
My work is done, I am free to leave. The vessels of your love (blood vessels) no longer have blocks, they are now free.
As soon as you feel better, get out and paint. Write positive loving quotes on canvas. A message from your soul.
It knows. And this has given you the belief and trust …and to let go of your past beliefs. Write some quotes." (Here are some ideas)

"Only when facing your worst fears,
do you know your inner strength."

"Focus on your vision
Feel it in every pore
Let your spine tingle
With trust and love"

"Just breathe and relax"

"The angels have your back"

A few days after calling them, St George's neurosurgery department phone us back and tell Dave my consultant appointment date and that the surgeon will be Timothy Jones. The appointment is a few days away - Tuesday. I don't get it. I have not seen a single person who can tell me anything concrete about what they are wanting to do to me, yet I am on an urgent waiting list for a brain operation. I am so confused. Terrified. Don't they realise that we know nothing apart from 'I need an operation ASAP'?

Each day I seem to swing the full pendulum of emotions. From believing I will have a spontaneous remission and it will be smaller when they look at it again, to shaking and sobbing with fear - the enormity of what is happening weighing down every millimetre of my body and soul. At night I just need to be held and cry and cry. I cannot get comfortable, my neck and head constantly hurt. Not as extreme as before, but certainly not right either. I want someone to tell me it will be alright. But they cannot.

I have a period again and for the first time in over 4 months I don't get a headache with it, much less the blinding one where I can barely move... maybe as my body doesn't have to 'scream' to make me realise I have something I need to address urgently? As i now know.

Tuesday 3rd May. Journal entry.

> *"We thought I had the consultant appointment this afternoon, as I heard Dave say (and write down) Tuesday on the phone, but a letter arrives this morning saying Thursday 5th May. We call them to confirm, but it's not today, it's Thursday".*

I want to scream. I feel sick. I had built up all my worries and expected them to get some kind of answer today- to get any answer!...and now I have to wait another two bloody days!!! I can't cope with this. Arrgghhh!!!

3/5/16. Journal entry - (again writing to self)

"Ok tumour- what else do I need to know"

"That you have to rest each day. Honour yourself. Connect to the Grace and the God in you.
You can hear it now. You really understand. You believe. You are genuinely feeling happy and whole- even when the world would try and make you not. Instead of fear you now trust and feel love.
Keep focussing on being healed. You are healed. You are healing yourself
Jo, now you have that power in your heart, you really are able to change worlds.
I LOVE YOU SO MUCH
Xxx
♥"

Chapter 9 - Angel Cards

After finding out about the tumour, I look through some of my journals (not that I continuously write them, but do jot down feelings etc when I want to.) In the journal I made at Hollie's workshop just a couple of weeks ago I realise I added these quotes to it:

"The scariest moment is always just before you start" - Stephen King

"I try to turn my brain off and let my heart draw"

"It wasn't until I accepted myself just as I was in this moment, that I was free to change" - Carl Rogers

"All I have is all I need and all I need is all I have in this moment" - Byron Katie

"It is by finally showing your weakness that you become really strong" – Griet Op de Beeck

Plus the singular words: *"surrender", "love", "peace" and "soul"*

Oh! I think my soul knew that I would need these quotes.

I also emailed Tina who had said she would give me a free Angel Card reading when she was at the creative day with me, having asked her the question: 'What do I need to know to heal my tumour?'

Today I get her reply back:

"The first vertical row down of cards is usually the past however it can be the basis of the situation and I feel that is the case here; it is referring to the present. You are being advised to accept the situation - that you are in the process of healing and that everything is going to be okay. The second card tells you to trust your inner guidance, your gut feelings, and trust any repetitive signs, visions (in your mind's eye) or dreams. The card says "you know what to do". By listening to and following your inner wisdom you will receive new wonderful good health (abundance 'Treasure Chest' card). The Acceptance card (from Archangel Raphael Healing deck) gives you a prayer: "Dear God and Archangel Raphael, please help me accept that everything is going in the right direction."

The second vertical row shows me that you haven't been sleeping very well. Sleep, rest and time out including walks in nature are all very important for your healing. The Moon Cycles card comes to you from Archangel Haniel to advise you that the night prior to the full moon is the perfect time to do healing and cleansing work on yourself. The next full moon is on 21st May so the best evening for healing work such as prayers is on 20th May. This card can also be referring to hormonal cycles which can be upset by stress and lack of sleep. It may be worth getting your hormone levels checked as they may need balancing. The last card in this row is about manifestation and reminds you that thoughts and their associated feelings become things. It strongly advises that to heal think only about yourself as already healed and feel the gratitude of that. Close your eyes every day and see yourself as healed. Feel the joy of good vibrant health. Ask the Angels to help you.

The last row again recommends self-care: Relaxing, healing massage is recommended - aromatherapy massage with frankincense oil would be good for you. And angel therapy is recommended. This reading for example is a form of angel therapy and of course so is praying to your guardian angels and the healing angels, especially Archangel Raphael. Surrender your situation to the angels. Hand it to them and let them carry it for you. They are waiting for you to ask. Remember because of free will angels can't help you unless you ask. Pray also to the angels who are brilliant at clearing negative toxic energy such as anger and unforgiveness - Archangels Uriel, Metatron, Michael and also Indriel.

"Dear Archangel Raphael and angels, I accept health now. Knowing that my body is safe, that my immune system is strong and that my blood flows beautifully around my body is absolutely perfect. All my major organs including my brain are filled with angelic healing light as I affirm my body is whole. I am healed, I am well and healthy! And so it is!"

The last card in this row Waves of Prosperity is very similar to the Treasure Chest card we talked about above. It means that with self-care and angel therapy you will receive abundant good health."

I did draw 3 Angel tarot cards for you which told me that in your recent past you've been busy, busy busy! So the advice for self-care now makes sense. There is now, in the present, a need to balance your emotions. Have you met a new partner recently? Or are you in a relationship that could be leading to marriage? I ask because this Knight of Water card can also mean falling in love or wedding proposals. In your near future you are going to feel like moving on to something new, to something more meaningful because you will have grown both emotionally and spiritually. That could refer to a relationship or to your work.

Jumping cards
You received several jumping cards. More than I've ever had to date during a reading! Jumping cards are cards which fly out of the deck while shuffling and they are considered important cards carrying important messages for you from the angels. The angels felt there was more to tell you!

From the Archangel Raphael Healing deck you received two beautiful cards that gave me goose bumps (angel bumps): Prayer Works and Recovery. It was very clear instantly to me that Archangel Raphael is giving you the message that prayers do work, that prayers to God and the angels will be heard and will be answered by your recovery. So please pray every day to the angels Jo. These two cards give you two prayers, the first you need to complete yourself (so Archangel Raphael has given you a little homework ☺)

"Dear God and Archangel Raphael, thank you for hearing and answering my prayer of [ADD THE DETAILS OF YOUR PRAYER].

"Dear Archangel Raphael, thank you for holding my hand throughout my recovery upon the path of radiant health."

Two other jumping cards included: Counsellor and Spiritual Understanding. I feel some kind of counselling support is being recommended for you. A safe place where you can talk freely and express yourself. Your spiritual awareness is going to grow. Notice symbols that have meaning for you. Putting these together, spiritual based counselling/coaching would be great for you and your healing journey right now.

The last jumping card was from the Angel Tarot deck: Six of Air. This is also a beautiful card which gives you the message that everything is going to be okay. It says "Things are looking up! The end of a difficult situation." It also mentions that you may take a trip in the future."

As I read this, yet again, I just cry! It tells me I am healing, it tells me to trust, it tells me to trust repetitive signs! (I cannot tell you how many times I have seen 11:11 or repeat numbers now!) I do know what to do... I need this operation and to let go. I haven't been sleeping. Yes my hormonal cycles have been messed up (and giving me the severe headache warning signs.) It tells me I need to see myself as healed - exactly what I believe and have been doing. I have just brought Frankincense oil. And well the future prediction part I just cry over... this has got to be part of my recovery. Not just from the tumour, but from me.

Chapter 10 - Meeting my Neurosurgeon

It's finally the 5th. This afternoon I have my neurosurgery consultant appointment. I am petrified. I don't like Dr's. I don't agree with most of them. I think them not understanding my view is as scary as having an operation. I am worried I am going to get a consultant who ridicules my opinion yet I will have no option but to go along with what he says and wants me do to, or what drugs I have to take. I might have to fight inside myself the alternative knowledge I have or feel, versus the standard medical procedures that they will almost certainly offer. And how do I say no if I really feel something is wrong when they insist it is ok? And what happens if I am wrong all along? As after all I cannot afford to see a private holistic doctor.

Nicola comes over and does an amazingly relaxing Gaia healing session with me before I go. I am able to see beautiful purple and yellow swirling around before me when my eyes are shut. Think positive and trust...

So we leave, allowing an hour to get there, park and to get inside (not helped by me being super slow at moving now and we don't know exactly where the appointment is held inside the neurosurgery wing shown on their map) ...and of course we run into road works. They have closed the road in the direction we are travelling and so we get diverted through Wimbledon. The traffic isn't moving. I could walk faster - well if I could walk properly. We move one small road length in 30 minutes. It's a really warm spring day and as we are moving so slowly the car starts jolting, Dave is concerned it must be overheating or something. But we cannot stop as we have 15 minutes to get to our appointment – and Google maps still says the hospital is 15 minutes' drive away! Thankfully we are out of the worst of the queuing traffic. I put the car heater on maximum settings - both as full and hot as I can, to hopefully take away the heat from the engine and we just drive, hoping we don't have to stop for too long at any junctions. But the mixture of heat, the worry the car might stop, the fear of missing the appointment time totally and getting sent home, the fear of finally getting to see the consultant and find out what's actually happening… and I just panic. A full blown feel even dizzier, feel sick to the stomach, think I am going to faint, panic.

Great. I know what is happening and am trying to calm myself down, but it isn't working. In the middle of Wimbledon High Street some woman driving a car in the lane next to us shouts out her window if we know where St George's is… so we shout back for her to follow us. I am contemplating that if our car stops totally we just leave the car where it is and get in hers to get to the hospital. I need to get there. It feels like my life depends on it – maybe it does?

Thankfully we (both) arrive at St George's with the car still working and find a parking space quite easily. Dave gets me out and we attempt to walk into the neurology wing - not an easy task now at any rate, but helped even less by the fact I am sobbing myself silly and feeling so weak and shaky I need to lie down. We get to reception a few minutes late but they calmly tell us everyone is late today as apparently there is a big problem with the tube network and it is all but shut down, so not to worry. I cry again!

I walk to the toilet, take some rescue remedy and try to calm myself. It works for about 10 seconds as the sobs start up again and I just want to lie down. I find the biggest space in the waiting room that I can- away from other people, shut my eyes, listen to my meditation music on my i-pod (this comes everywhere with me now) and just continue to breathe. Breathe in, breathe out. This is about all I can manage right now. Yet if I listen inside I feel I am waiting to meet my executioner and for him to tell me how, where and when he is going to kill me…

Then a smiley face calls my name… and I get a happy handshake and welcome from Timothy Jones the neurosurgeon. Well he seems confident- so that's a positive! In his room he asks me to do some more of the neurological tests and asks when we have noticed the symptoms from. Badly - the last few months since December, more mildly... last year, maybe even the past few years. Could it be decades? My balance has been awful for so long- could it be this tumour? He tells us this type of tumour is really slow growing and can have been here for years...

Did I ever have any family members who had similar tumours, or anything else mysterious in my family history that anyone died from? No. He explains there is a genetic link to this type of tumour and 'if' it's genetic, while I could be the first in the family to get it, there is normally someone who had a similar problem. But I am of the right age - early 40's- when it is the non-genetic type and just occurs seemingly randomly. I ask could it have been as I fell and hit this same area a few year ago. No. Could it be linked to EMF's? No - it is not a radiation induced type of tumour.

He then tells us about what he has to do during the operation... I just feel even more numb and tearful again and can barely take anything in. I can barely breathe, let alone listen. If I asked him what he told me I am sure it would be very different, but mainly all I remember is the fact this tumour bleeds - and often badly - as it is made up of blood vessels. I will most likely need a blood transfusion. They would have some blood ready in theatre and that it's ok as St George's has a blood bank on site if they need any more. (I think this is supposed to reassure me... it doesn't - I just have ghastly images of all my blood draining from me while they try and get more in.) They have to cut and seal around the outside of it, slowly; and they cannot just scoop into it or it will just bleed uncontrollably - and it can then cause you to bleed to death! I think he said something about if it does bleed they will just have to scoop quickly and remove it all to seal it as soon as they can, but they don't want to do this. Oh ... and that the operation has a 1 in 1000 chance of bleeding to death during it ... my brain temporarily switched off again at this point and another bucket load of tears got released!

I think he says something about if it all gets removed ok, then I will have a normal lifespan and life again after. Albeit I will have some side effects from the operation but I will have to live with them as they cannot be avoided. I will still be alive. But also that I might well hate him for doing the operation as I have about a 5% chance of a bigger problem happing during surgery, such as a stroke or similar damage. But if he doesn't do it I would hate him more- as I **will** have a stroke or something and then basically die within a few months!! Ok. 5%... that means 95% chance of it being ok. But 5% chance of being totally screwed up... I didn't even know I had a tumour 2 weeks ago. Now I need urgent surgery or I will basically die. I can't take this in.

They will put some kind of acrylic 'plate' over the piece of skull they will remove at the back, I will also need the front of my head drilled to put a drainage tube in - to remove excess fluid and therefore protect my brain from the pressure during the operation. They aim to just cut straight up the centre back of my head a few inches starting from my neck - I should barely have a visible scar after as it will mostly be in my hair line and they only shave off the hair near where they cut.

The insides of my elbows and hands are literally crawling, it's like when your nerves have all gone mad from hearing someone scratching their nails down a chalk board. I can't cope listening. I want it all written down and to be able to read one sentence at a time, when I can understand and take it in - slowly. Take my time to comprehend it. I don't do hospitals, I don't do surgery ... or blood ... or needles ... or drips ... or drainage tubes or even looking at or reading about it. It's gross! Even watching a TV programme like 'Casualty' makes me feel the emotions of actually being there and I feel nauseous and panicky. Not that I watch most films or TV dramas – as they affect me far too much!

I ask can this type of tumour ever shrink naturally and he says no, so I question is a hemangioblastoma different to 'normal' brain tumour types as I know I have read of others shrinking them even when stage 4, with natural treatments. He categorically says nothing natural will shrink a stage 4 brain tumour, or we would all know about it.

I think I add that I normally use various alternative therapies and don't even take normal pain killers and he talks about alternatives or complementary therapies being great for when you can do complementary things to help alongside medical treatment. I don't even want to start on the fact I believe in energy healing etc, as while a part of me knows all sorts is possible, I don't know if this type of tumour is ever able to heal, and I know I have to trust him (and not piss him off too much!) I guess he can tell that I am normally not open to medical treatment as he then also tells me that I will have to take the medication the doctors prescribe. I agree. I know I have no choice.

I really cannot remember what he says after this point, but know it is something along the lines of 'was I always like this?' and me saying I just had a panic attack getting here and yes I am often anxious but no, not like this. Him saying that I needed to try and relax as I would have a better outcome than if I am stressed and that they expect me to stay in hospital for about a week. He also points out that I will feel 'really' dizzy after the operation. That it won't be easy and that dizziness may last for 3 months or so, but will eventually settle down.

I know at some point I told him I don't want surgery at full moon (as I have been told you can bleed more then and well he has just told me this tumour bleeds more than most and I don't need another risk...) and that he would contact us later with the date, but it wouldn't be before 14th May (the date of our son Zach's 18th birthday) but most likely before the end of May.

He asks am I still driving, to which I answer "No, I stopped a few weeks back when the dizziness became too much" and he says I will not be able to drive again for 6 months after the operation as the DVLA have a ban on driving for that long after you have a drain put in your head during brain surgery. Although he says it may be longer if I have any side effects or have a fit. Great! But, I guess, at least they think I will be able to drive again. Be normal.

I leave his room and he gives both Dave and I a handshake - and all I remember thinking is he has short solid fingers and they are going to be inside my skull! ... Well I guess they are less wobbly when operating.

I leave the neurology department and hospital, walking along holding Dave's arm just breaking down and crying bucket loads...I am vaguely aware the area is full of people, but I don't care who sees me. I don't even care if there is a child I am scaring by my crying so much. In fact I don't even know if any children are there as I am blind to everything. I just don't care. I don't give a shit. I've just been told I could bleed to death during the operation. My skull needs opening. I'm panicking again. I feel hollow. The world seems slow and unreal... all the people in the hospital look happy- how? I don't get it? The planet has just stopped.

We get back in the car and I think Mr Jones and anyone else who saw me must just think I am insane. I feel it.

As we get in the car Dave tells me that he thinks the car was mucking around as the oil in some part of the car was low and the heat expanded it and made it worse - hence why it was driving oddly. I don't know what he is on about, I don't really care.

Although thankfully the car seems to be working alright now. I just want to go home. I want to go to bed and cry in privacy. Pretend this isn't happening. I take some more aconite for the panic, and just sit there sobbing all my fear away and text a couple of people for some support...

5th May 17:47. Text to Nicola as I am in car.

> *"Really screwed up...started with car overheating, road works and a panic attack...ended with the fact its ok technically to operate on- but this type bleeds and likelihood is I need a blood transfusion and you can bleed to death ... No words apart from terrified as I feel so negative and I need loads of medication etc etc"*

What do I say to anyone? I cannot even say the info to myself yet without crying. I don't even think I have taken it in nor admitted it to myself. Can I just hide and let others do it? Do I need to write a letter to each of the kids in case I die? But I don't want to write it as then it's like I believe I will be that 1 in 1000. But if I don't, and I die, then I haven't told them what they really mean to me and how much I love them. Just as they are. All very different. Faults and all. But amazing, beautiful and oh so talented, and I am so proud of them. To see who they changed into, from those precious new-born's that I brought into this world...

I'm working the odds out in my head ... At the kids' old secondary school there must be close to 2000 kids... so that means 1 or 2 of them if they all had this operation would die, and 100 would have a serious problem after ... that's too many. Suddenly the percentage risk seems more.

Oh fucking shut up!!! ... Sometimes I wish my thoughts would just stop ... Shut up and stop fucking tormenting me.

Chapter 11 - Terrified Acceptance

I listen over and over to mediation CDs, Abraham Hicks work, positive spontaneous healing stories and keep asking and asking the Angels to hold me as I need them here with me now for comfort and to keep me safe during the operation.

I see online many stories of people healing naturally from all sorts - or as Dr's call them 'spontaneous remissions' - and see many stories of people healing from cancer or tumours using alternative things. People have told me their stories of how they healed when I asked for advice on a natural health group and I know and have met people who have healed themselves in the past. I have read and seen many cases from people who were even classed as terminal cases leaving hospices and going into remission – years ago. I fully believe this is possible. Totally 100% believe that the doctors are not always right and there is both lots you can do yourself in changing circumstances, diet and emotions and that there is also something much bigger too, including that you get what you need to be able to grow, and that we are all connected.

But my ego mind is feeling totally torn as the surgeon categorically said you cannot heal naturally from this type of tumour. Is it even physically possible for anything to reduce a hemangioblastoma? Is it a bit like saying I am going to grow a new limb? Would I just be dreaming that I can? I don't want to die as I think I believe in this and choose to wait...

6th May. Written in journal, just after I wake.

> *"OK. So yesterday I saw surgeon, and got told my tumour is completely possible to heal from – but it's risky in the fact it's the blood vessels and that it bleeds. I'm scared.*

Scared of dying of course, but scared of blood transfusion(s), medications, not being well, not being in control, seeing my kids scared, having to totally give in and surrender to others and trust.

I normally only 'trust myself' and yet I have to let that go. It's above me now.
Yes, I can trust that if I had more time (and found out far earlier), I could shrink it. But in 2 weeks I either need a miracle or to just let go. I need to work out that I 'can' let go of this and sorting it and yet not let go of life too. I guess I always equated them to the same thing. But they are not.

I still feel in shock at times, but am slowly getting back to the fact that life is still going. The world has just re-wound for me, but everyone else is the same.
Innocent. Free. Happy. Something I have never really been for a very long time.
But something I know that once I am over this I will never let go of again.
Each day is a blessing and I needed to realise that.

I CAN do what I desire, I need to be strong... and trust."

As ever, I just cry. A strange 'I can't cope with this' flood of tears but somehow they help in releasing the fears. Helping me know what I need to do.

I realise I need support... I need others to help support me. I can't do it alone and so I reach out with a post on Facebook to all my friends.

Posted on Facebook.

"Long post alert... but please read
I wasn't going to tell all of you, but then decided that I need to be true to me and I need some support

Anyway I found out a couple of weeks ago that I have a brain tumour - a cerebellar hemangioblastoma- slightly different to most brain tumours as it's in the blood vessels in the cerebellum (the back of the head)

The Dr's want to remove it and say it will 'never' shrink... (which I don't believe) but I feel I do probably need it removed, but I want to see if i can shrink it a bit and make it easier to remove etc... But to someone who has tried to live as naturally as I can, this is a big head fuck. A serious operation, the medication, the fact i will almost definitely need a blood transfusion...

So basically- I need your support please.... please can you send me any healing vibes, pray, send any loving support, or just think me good wishes. (and no negative x) and well if I can reduce it and the symptoms I will be immensely grateful!
❤
I feel that the wind has been taken from beneath me and I need others to hold me up for a while...
xxx   thank you ❤ *xxx"*

I am overwhelmed with the love sent back to me. People just saying a few words to let you know they care means so much. They see me as healed, even if I can't right now.

6th May 17.00. Text to Nicola.

> *"Am felling lots better than yesterday afternoon! Still more than a bit scared when I think of the op, but can find the peace within again.*
> *It's like everything is magnified...my love for people...even those just being kind to me and I don't know iyswim- and things...*
> *Just everything is so raw and delicate...*
> *Also, surgeon said they would not do another scan...I just need to trust that if I am making it smaller it is a good thing*
> *And you have no idea how much it means to have your thoughts and healing...I know I'm emotional...but its huge* "

That evening Dave and Zach are playing a gig at a local pub. Mum says she is coming over to 'babysit' me and then Adam says he wouldn't mind going to watch for a while. I need to get out - I feel I have been imprisoned for months and need to get out and try and switch off. We decide to go for a while. Mum drives me to the pub. I am vaguely ok when I am sitting in the car, but then there are road works outside the pub and we have to park a little further back than normal. We all walk up the road thinking we can get in one way, then cannot as the pathway is totally blocked at the end, so we have to walk back and in another way. Just doing this and I am exhausted and feel sick. This was a mistake, but we have now collected Adam and, well, we are here.

I walk in the pub and sit down. I don't know if there was, amazingly, a spare seat as the place was packed or I just took it, but I had to sit down. Walking past the PA speakers seemed so loud, but even sitting at the back of the room it just seems to be turned up too much. More than I can stand. I put in ear plugs. Then I realise that even the vibrations of the music are hurting my head. It is just too much for me to cope with. I want to go home.

I sit there thinking I am going to hold everything together and attempting to talk to a friend who knows and is offering his sympathy - although I am struggling to hear anything but the music far too loudly in my head. But also know that I cannot keep up this pretence of being normal anymore, I can't and don't want to pretend all is ok. I feel shaky inside. Sick to the core. Silently scared and screaming. Thankfully about 4 songs after we arrived it is the end of the first set, Dave comes over and I tell him I cannot cope and need to leave now, so I walk past the band, wave goodbye to Zach as I try not to cry again and get Dave to walk me back to the car. Oh well it was worth a try- it just didn't work. In fact it failed miserably. Will I ever be able to listen to music loud again without my head feeling like it will explode? Will I ever be able to see my son, or husband, play in a band again and be able to enjoy it?

I have someone (whose support, advice and opinion I have previously respected) who is telling me how they are treating a family member's tumour in a kidney and that I should look at alternatives or maybe just wait and see for a while. I listen, and the holistic part of me somewhat agrees; but I also want to scream 'you have two fucking kidneys, if you fuck up with this you can go back to the mainstream doctors and surgery, get the kidney removed totally and still have another one he can live on. I only have one brain, I have fluid expanding around it which could cause serious problems if it gets any worse and no second chance.'

Not to mention I can't afford to keep getting MRI scans to track progress, and the NHS won't do them for free if I don't follow their path. Then there are the slightly important facts that I can't even see the computer properly to research things nor even look at the TV screens from a distance. That I cannot walk properly - or even think properly. I can't see my face well enough to even attempt to put make up on, I can't even have a shower without Dave there to help me and it's totally exhausting when I do. It's not like I have a tumour and yet I am still able to continue my life. Moving from bed, to sofa, to garden recliner, to toilet and back is not a life. I am existing. Just.

Somewhere in this I connect with my body and realise that 'I' need the operation, and accept it. I am still terrified, but I finally accept I need it done.

I get told the date of my operation - 25th May, and the pre op assessment - 10th May. It's not long.

9th May. Text to Alison

> "It's so blooming tiring when you are unable to do much…yes it's got to the point that I need the op- as much as that 'isn't me' ☹ I want to be able to do things again… went to a Ransom gig Friday with Mum and Adam, but just couldn't hack the noise, vibration or even being there…was getting more and more panicky ☹ had to go home after about 4 songs (at half time) …it's like I cannot be me anymore… roll on op…"

Its pre op day … no road works or delays this time, but I still end up getting there a quivering mess of jelly. Not helped by the fact I can't walk properly and even doing so for a short while makes me visibly shaky and it's not just anxiety. Thankfully they have a whole pre op centre that is separate to the main hospital and so not only do I not have to walk in the main part of the building, it's also just off the car park and less far to go. We sit in the waiting room and I manage to fill in my basic contact details. Even writing in capitals is so hard now - I feel I am having to spell out each letter in a word and also getting letter shapes wrong. After handing the form back I get called through by the nurse and she does some simple height, weight and blood pressure type checks. I only weigh 7 stone 13! I know I have had no appetite to eat much for weeks but this is ridiculous I must have lost just over a stone within in a few months. I've lost 7lb since I was weighed at the MRI, a couple of weeks ago. She checks my heart rate and it is too fast... I think I could have told them that! How could they expect it to be anything different? - I hate hospitals, I hate bleeps, I can hear ambulance sirens going past and I am sitting here getting my brain operation details and discussing what blood type I am for the likelihood of needing a blood transfusion! So I need an ECG - which is all fine- and then go to see the craniotomy nurse.

Charlotte is lovely and reassuring. She says yes it's ok to feel terrified and most people are when they know they need brain surgery. But to them it is a daily procedure. Daily. She speaks to several people each week all having various forms of brain surgery. Several of them who are having brain tumours removed are generally healthy younger people (in 30s or 40s) and she now gets a few of these each month- and her voice wanders as she seemingly queries why the numbers are increasing. (Oh wow... I am so sure many of these will be linked to EMF's -electromagnetic field- and the fact that so many people have a mobile phone all but glued to their head...)

She is happy that everything is normal - I normally eat well, I don't drink or smoke, am not asthmatic or diabetic - and so should have no problems with the op. She says she will email all the details over to me, tells me that I will have to stay in hospital for around 5-9 days. 7 being about average. I ask her is there 'any' chance I will come home before this, so I can prepare myself for how long I need to stay, and she clearly says "no, it will be 5 days minimum". I am told to continue with my meditation CDs and anything that will help relax me, as if I am calmer it will speed up my healing, prevent more complications and reduce the time I will need to stay in hospital. Just before I leave, she retakes my blood pressure and pulse and it is back to normal.

I also apparently need to stop taking any supplements from now as they don't want any to interfere with the medication I will need during and after the operation. I query with what I am taking but the only thing I can continue is my food level vitamin C.

10th May. Text to Nicola

> "Felt like stressed crap again this morning before pre op… then after talking to craniotomy nurse calmed down (and got my heartbeat back to normal speed!) she was saying there are more and more 'youngish healthy people' having brain tumours… (I am sure mobile and EMFs etc…) and basically she was happy I am ok for op x
> Helped reassure me it's 'normal' to feel scared, but I will be ok. And they are there to support me etc was told to do as much meditation and calming stuff as possible… which I know inside x
> I am ok ish until I get near a hospital and then I seem to lose it…
>
> I weighed 7st 13 today!! I know I haven't felt hungry but I have lost 7lbs in 2.5 weeks ☹ (and had been almost 9 stone last summer) nurse said I should try and fatten myself up a bit…not sure how when I don't feel like eating much"

The next day Roan has a dentist appointment to get a baby tooth that is stuck pulled out and as much as I know he hates dentists and I want to be there for him, I can't even consider going as I feel so awful. So he gets given his arnica and aconite tablets and Dave takes him, with strict instructions to sit on the end of the dentist's chair and reassure him. They soon return with the tooth removed and a smile, while I am still in exactly the same place on the sofa. I'm failing at 'Mum' duties too.

It's the same with his Judo and rock climbing classes that week - I feel barely able to respond, let alone with any enthusiasm. It seems my neck movements are reducing almost every day, now I cannot even move my head to look to the side of me. Everything takes so long to do and is so controlled. And my headaches are seemingly returning - albeit not as painful as before.

I feel like total crap as its Zach's 18th birthday and I can't do a thing apart from wish him Happy Birthday. I cannot buy a card or make a cake (well I ordered some 'birthday treat' food online- does that count?) I can't help with anything, can't take him out. Can't turn around when family come in with presents. Cannot do anything to celebrate or make it a memorable day. I just am stuck here on the sofa barely able to move without a headache watching endless episodes of Big Bang Theory on TV and falling asleep!

14th May. Text to Dave in evening (as out at gig)

> "I am in same place on sofa- but ok if I am here, head shitty if I move still ☹ "

15th May. When I finally get up this morning (after a night of seemingly constant headaches, neck pain and ear ringing) I laugh at myself in the mirror and take a picture... I post this on Facebook.

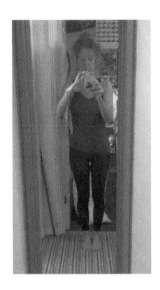

"Well you have to laugh sometimes...
Anyone want to join me on the brain tumour diet? You can
lose up to 7lbs in 2 weeks, not feel like eating, see your
bones in your hips are higher than your belly, have thigh
gaps and have arms smaller than your kids?
Although the side effects are: you cannot walk too well,
occasionally have an evil headache and you feel shite... But
hey many people do that each time after they go out !! ☺
Be real ❤ ❤ xx"

Another day of doing nothing but worry, and yet trying to trust.

Chapter 12 - Hell and Prayers

16th May. Second night of being awake with headaches and slightly concerning high pitched ear ringing so we decide to go to St George's A&E and get it checked, hopefully I will be able to get some kind of painkiller that works. As all the kids are still asleep we decide to leave them there and just wake Zach enough to tell him where we are going.

We get there, slowly, wobbly and with lots of tears and laughter at how ridiculous this is, and get seen by the triage, then have to wait on the slightly uncomfortable but sanitary metal seating. Then some guy walks round saying that they are filming '24 hours in A&E' and would I be happy being on there? I ask what the hell that is and get told it's a TV programme. Um yeah right... I am sitting here probably more fucked up as I have ever been in my life: I look puffy from sobbing, have tied up hair that I have not been able to wash today or even yesterday, cannot sit up straight, know I have a brain tumour and that I need a major operation next week, can't speak straight as it hurts to think, and am in pain ...but you want to ask me if I give my permission for someone else to watch my torture? Fuck off.

We get told that 'if' they use any footage with us in the picture, then they will blank our faces out so we are not recognisable. I don't give a shit about just having a fuzzy face - I think the whole idea of filming other people's pain is sick. If it was for doctors, nurses or even planning or training purposes, then yes I get it; but for this warped enjoyment - it just shouldn't even be considered. Plus if anyone we know saw a scrawny ill looking redhead and a bloke with long blond hair they would know it was us even if they blanked it out so you couldn't see our damn faces! It's my bloody tumour (literally) and I don't want anyone to see me and feel sorry for me - I am trying to only attract healing and loving thoughts. So I sit here sticking my fingers up at the camera every time it moves it our direction- thankfully whoever was watching and recording it seemed to get the message and moved the camera elsewhere.

As I sit here still swearing as to how fucked up it is to video in A&E and how anyone would ever want to watch others pain - my name gets called. They tell me I need to have a cannula put in my arm and they take some blood and a while later we get called to a cubicle area where they will get a neurosurgeon. Great! Another fucking camera and microphone dangling over my head... roll on more rude signs and comments at it and blocking my face with my cardigan over my head. Even if I am sitting here and they are not actually filming me, I don't want someone watching me. It's supposed to be private. That's why they have curtains around the cubicle. You wouldn't have a camera and microphone in a toilet would you? Would they be allowed to show 24 hours in a public toilet?!

The neurosurgeon, and trainee doctors, turn up and one asks me, yet again, to do all the basic tests - and still it seems the only one I cannot do is the heel to toe test. I try and say to the doctors that I don't have a problem with them and sorry for being rude. Although I am not sure what they think of me as I seem to be putting in a swear word into every sentence - purely so they won't ever use any footage of me on TV - and I do point it out to them how disgusting I find it having a camera in here more than once.

Text to Adam- 11.43

> *"Up at St Georges, went to A&E as head still shite* ☹ *stuck here for now waiting... and if you see a blurry figure on 24hrs in A&E it's me- and Dad!*
> *Refused to sell my soul to TV – esp for free entertainment – how fucking awful!!! Why would anyone find it entertaining??*

(Adam replies- K finds it interesting – from nurses point of view)
Well tell her if there is a blurry pair of yetis it's us! They said
we could still be filmed but they would blur our faces...
Good job with the way I look at moment eh?! ☺

(Would they have paid you to be filmed?)

"Didn't offer- but it was the only way they would be! About
10K would do it. They can even do the op if enough for a
house!!
Is A&E prog live? Camera turned the other way now- don't
think it likes V signs ☺
And there is a bloody microphone hanging over my head!"

I get sent off for a CT scan - great, more radiation, but do I have any choice? I am sitting outside the x-ray room at the end of A&E sobbing. There is a secondary school age boy with a cast on his foot along with his mum sitting next to me. When he goes in the room she kindly asks "Are you ok?" and I just start sobbing "No, not really" explaining I have a brain tumour that needs removing and I am terrified. She asks me would I mind if she prays for me... No, I don't mind.

So for the next few minutes she holds my hands in hers and prays out loud for Jesus to heal me. Now the word Jesus I don't really use or understand the meaning of, but the rest of her wording and her intention I did. Totally. She was praying to see me fully healed and well after this. Praying to release all my fears and to give me strength. It was like she spoke and released all my fears, sending me full love for several minutes and yet I didn't even know her!

At some point after she stopped praying, another woman walked past, grabbed a tissue from the dispenser, handed it to me and said "Here you go. We are all one" as she continued on her way... and I sobbed some more. The woman's son returned from his scan and she chatted about what ward I was going to be on and when my operation was. I replied I don't know which ward, but I think there are only two wards in neurosurgery and the op is next Wednesday the 25th. She said she was having to return with her son the day after so she would call in and see how I was. It is odd to describe meeting a stranger and it being a totally loving kind encounter, but that is all I can describe it as.

I never got her name. But thank you, thank you so much. Xxxx

So off I go to have my scan done - thankfully CT scans are quick, as I couldn't lay still for long.

I walk back to Dave sitting in the cubicle and the nurse comes in to say they want to give me morphine... great. I hate drugs, I hate being spaced out... but I am going to have to get used to them - so here goes. Yuck... there must have been as much pink aspartame, E numbers and fake cherry flavour in that as there was morphine. I joke that I have just had my last 10 years of E numbers and sweeteners in one dose of pink drug, but not sure the nurse understands! I try and drown the disgusting sickly sweet taste with my now cold bottle of nettle tea.

A little while later they say they are moving me to another area - Clinical Dependency Unit ... so I walk arm in arm with Dave, him keeping me walking straight while we follow the nurse. I am very loudly declaring "I'm fully pissed now, I walk drunk normally, and now I'm properly drunk as I'm pissed on morphine!"

For some reason they don't have cameras in the CDU...

Chapter 13 - Music Keeping Me Sane

Text to Adam

> *"Am here for a while (well hours not days!) as waiting for CT scan results. Been given liquid morphine so fully pissed now!! And cameras have gone from here...*
> *Had my jacket over my head and tapping to Muse. Now stuck on a fucking chair ☹ and I really want to sleep"*

We get some chairs to sit on while they wait for a bed to become available. We have 3 chairs in a row in a gap opposite the toilet. I want to lie down, but cannot, and try various positions of trying to lean on Dave- but nothing seems comfortable.

We ask the nurses can we get any food and she tells us we have missed the meals, but there is a canteen and shop. So Dave goes to get us some lunch from the shop and comes back with the only gluten free option he could find - a cheese sandwich. Oh joy! Like I was already feeling ill enough without stomach ache too. But I'm hungry, so cheese sandwich it is.

And we wait...

For another few hours...

14.56. Text to Nicola

> *"When waiting for scan a woman waiting for her son asked how I was and I said it was a BT. She asked could she pray for me, so she did- saying similar to what I had but about God & Jesus, not Angels x and another woman walked past and got me a tissue and said 'we are all one!'* ♥

There is far more love than I realised before and its
everywhere!
I know something good has got to come from this x ❤
Just wanted to say to someone who understands xxxx"

Text to Adam.

"I'm just tired and pissed. Was talking bollox earlier, now
just sleepy..."

I finally get a bed in the CDU around 5.30pm and half clonk out on it. Dave goes back to the shop to find more food and there isn't any. The best he can find is a gluten free loaf of bread and some hummus. When he comes back we ask for a toaster and the nurses say they don't have one as they are deemed a fire risk. So I get to dunk some disgusting, crumbly, fake bread into a pot of cold hummus. I manage about 2 slices and it's more than enough.

Text to Alison.

"Needed scan 1ish, and only had a chair to sit on until after 5
(not good when barely slept for 2 nights) In CDU"

The nurses then tell me I will be staying in tonight as the surgeon isn't there to check my CT scan, and I definitely have fluid showing on my brain. I may stay in CDU but they are trying to get me a bed in a neurology ward. Dave tells me he needs to go home as he is exhausted and needs some sleep, and food. I tell him not to worry about bringing me anything. I will sleep in my leggings fine and can have a shower tomorrow. I have my phone, iPod and charger. I get a hug and he goes.

21.16. Text to Adam

*"Staying in this eve ☹ no one to see scan and precaution ...
I'm not good by myself....*
*Only on paracetamol and ibruprofen atm, but the happy pills
are at the ready*
*Actually it was a happy squirt! ☹ ...of disgusting aspartame
cherry flavour morphine!! My e no intake this decade just
trebled!!!!*
*And no organic, or wheat free food, not even toasters or
anything!! ☹"*

About 30 minutes after Dave leaves the nurse comes in to say I
cannot eat anything else now as they might be doing the operation
tomorrow morning... What the fuck?! I was only coming in here for
pain killers. I haven't even said goodbye to the kids - although how
the hell would I say goodbye to the kids? Dave isn't here and is too
shattered to come back. I am scared - big time. And they might
operate tomorrow morning... I just sit, sob and shake. I want to talk
to someone, but there is no one to walk to. Once again it's a
seemingly unreal nightmare. The nurse who tells me she is taking
me up to the neurology ward later (they found a bed) eventually
sees what a state I am in and talks to me about her needing an
operation recently and how awful she felt beforehand, and that I
really am in the best hands here. I still have to wait for the bed to
be ready and so just sit, shake and cry. Alone. I want someone to
hold me- anyone. And yet there is no one, no one can rescue me
from this. I have to face it...

Text sent to a few friends

*"Shitting a brick as I am going up to neurology... and said nil
by mouth in case..."*

I get stuck in a wheelchair and taken upstairs to the neurosurgery ward. It's odd even being moved in a wheelchair as my brain can't seem to keep up with the movement and it all feels a bit of a blur. I remember the porter and nurse both talking to me saying they did 12 hour shifts and my amazement that they expect anyone to work for twelve hours in a row, especially as they are supposed to be looking after people. How do they cope? They get used to it was the reply.

As I enter the ward everything is dark and the other five patients are seemingly asleep, or attempting to be. Although I then feel I am waking them all up as I get questioned by the nurses and one of the registrars comes in. Not to mention that I am still a little off my face on morphine and nervous tension so probably rather loud! The registrar tells me she is pleased to see how well I look, as from the scan she thought I would be in a worse state, (How do I take that?!) and she is reassured from seeing me. So they won't be doing the operation first thing tomorrow and I can eat again. My scan will be reassessed by Mr Jones in the morning and they will tell me what is happening as they may still bring the operation forwards. She continues to tell me that St George's is one of the best hospitals in the country to have brain surgery and that she would chose to have it here if she ever needed it. It sort of helps calm me that I am in the best place. I am given some high dose steroids to reduce the inflammation in my brain. I take them without even questioning or looking at the side effects (so unlike me) ... but know I have no choice.

Text to Dave.

> "Am ok for night ♥ been seen by a surgeon and can eat again.
> 'Might' move it forwards but possibly not. Calming down now! ♥"

The ward seems like something from a horror film. People are groaning and making odd noises, a couple of them keep farting, the woman next to me obviously cannot speak properly as she seems to be only able to make noises that resemble words when the nurses ask her something, and the older woman opposite looks like she is dying in the bed. She is seemingly asleep yet doing a funny rolling things with her hands, reaching for something invisible in the air above her- which reminds me of how my Grandad was when he was asleep just before he died. I pull my curtains to try and block out the sights and lights, and turn my iPod up so the earphones drown out the noises. Thankfully (as I know how much I need it) I brought the iPod charger with me!

I barely manage to sleep. I feel like I am wired with some drug or the stress, am struggling with all the bleeps, noises, lights and as soon as I think I am about to fall asleep a nurse comes to check me. I do almost sleep for a couple of hours at around 3am - I think when the exhaustion finally hit. In the morning I ask one of the doctors could the medication they gave me last night have made me feel buzzy, wired and unable to sleep and get told that yes the steroids can stop you from sleeping which is why they normally only give them in the day if they can, and yes some people get that 'wired feeling' from them. Why did I already know that?!

17th May 06.51. Text to Dave

> *"Am wide awake! They start doing checks at 5.30am when the light comes in! Hope you all slept ok? They said Mr Jones will be round this morning to discuss- will try to not just sob at him this time! But registrar last night was reassuring it's a 'routine' op again when I asked x*
>
> *Last night - head was good- only a couple of times it twinged. But they gave me steroids before I went to sleep.*

I was a good girl and am leaving the meds to Dr's and me to try and stay calm and trust x

Slept listening to music until about 3 (getting used to the freaky noises) and then crashed until 5.30 x They still 'might' do op tomorrow, and I need you here if they tell me xxx"

Well, although I haven't been properly told, from everyone's comments it seems I am staying in here ... I am staying plugged into my iPod with the meditation CDs on it. I need it to calm me down and keep me sane. I need to focus on calm and trust and not the reality and fear that hits as soon as I start to listen to the sounds of this place. I don't know what to describe it as for someone who is has sensory sensitivity- except torture?

Dave arrives early (out of visiting hours) with my clothes, toiletries and some rhubarb crumble Calla has made. I had missed breakfast as they said I was still nil by mouth then- and they don't have anything wheat free in the kitchens! I manage to eat most of it, although after I finish they say to not eat again until they have confirmed I am not having the operation later this afternoon! What? Are they trying to send me insane? They cannot keep doing this, the lack of control is just making me even more terrified.

The nurses move me to another ward, which seems to have older women on it that have all had, or need, spinal surgery. It's not as intense as the other ward. I am allowed to eat again, it won't be today. Surgery will likely be on Wednesday morning.

Dave leaves as my Mum is coming in with Roan at visiting time.

12.56. Text to Dave.

> *"Saw consultants (not Mr Jones) and still looking at*
> *tomorrow, but only if there are no urgent cases in today.*
> *Going to try and get some sleep now- and so scared x"*

Roan comes in with my Mum and instantly sits on the bed with me...he looks scared and I try and reassure him that everyone in the ward is ok and are getting better. But mainly we just hug in silence. He brings me the cuddly toy rabbit that a friend bought me recently when they found out I had a tumour and we discuss that I will cuddle my rabbit and he can cuddle his one (that looks very similar) at home and it will be the hug we cannot have while I am in here. We discuss that he knows what homeopathy to take when he needs it. I had written down at home a few remedies and the reasons he might want to take them if he was feeling he was missing me, or scared or his tooth was again hurting. I don't know what to say to him. I am trying to keep positive and hide my fears, but scared something will happen and this is the last time I will see him, or the last time I see him without having a disability. We talk about things he has been doing at home, small talk. The hug seems to say it all without saying a word - I hope he understands. He and Mum leave and I pull my curtains around to cry.

Dave returns at some point after they have left, again alone. We sit not knowing what to say, it's all been said several times before. I make him sit on the bed with me, even though he is not supposed to, as I need a cuddle. The nurses confirm that they are still planning to operate tomorrow, but only if there are no emergencies and so although it's planned we won't know for sure until the morning. We try and talk about feeling better once this lump has gone, once I stop feeling dizzy and drunk.

He takes this picture of me and later posts it on my and his Facebook wall saying:

"My operation has now been scheduled for 12 noon tomorrow (18-05-16). Please think positive thoughts for me around this time, thank you so much"

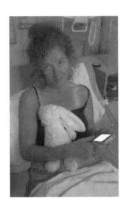

My mum brings Calla back here in the evening, we chat about her having to take a GCSE today when she really wasn't in the mood and said she could have fallen asleep at the desk. Mum also tells me that my aunt spoke to her and they moved my uncle to a hospice today! My aunt is happy that he is getting better care than he was in hospital, but going to a hospice? I can't deal with this right now. I can't see my uncle, I can't support my aunt or cousins, or do anything but send my love. I haven't been able to see any of them since he found out he was ill. The doctors feel he is now very terminally ill and possibly won't live much longer. Why does one person live and another die? Both of us are severely ill. Do they know they are really dying? How do I know I am not dying too? Does the soul know that this is the end and is somehow OK with it? I don't feel ready to die. But does anyone? I cannot deal with this now. It's too close, too raw. Yet I just silently think it, I daren't even say it to myself out loud, let alone to anyone else.

As they are here the second surgeon who will be operating on me comes round and confirms with me that the operation is scheduled for 12 noon tomorrow. Although I am third in surgery, which may make it slightly later, the other two operations are not expected to overrun. He explains the surgery procedure and risks again to me, this time all written down clearly. I have to sign each part. That I agree to the procedure and the risks involved, the fact there will be students there, if they can take photographs or videos if needed, that they can use the tissue for research etc. I am sobbing and laughing at the fact I am signing this shit... like I have any choice that they might struggle to take some membrane away from my skull and they need to do things slightly differently! They will have my skull opened- I won't exactly get to choose! As he finishes he asks if I have any further questions or concerns. "Yes", I laugh, "can I just ask you not to get drunk tonight as you are operating on my head tomorrow!" He looks seriously at me. I don't know that he sees the funny side of it, so I apologise and say I have to joke about it or I cannot cope.

Calla and Mum go, and again I am left to my own thoughts and fears.

20.43. Text to everyone.

> *"Have op at 12 noon tomorrow... please send all healing, prayers and ease of removal for then* ❤
> *Thank you all for caring- you have all helped so much* xxx
> ❤ ❤ xxx"

And added on this same text to a few....

> *"I am going to ask Angels to protect me and surgeons tomorrow too ...it's got to be magnified if others do it too ❤ ❤"*

Chapter 14 - Operation Brain Tumour

I don't even attempt to sleep and just try to relax. I play games on my phone while also listening to music and my meditations, trying to switch off and vaguely get comfortable in the bed. I must have moved the angle of the bed up and down one hundred times- trying to get comfortable with a tender neck, solid bed and rubbish pillow- while at the same time concerned I am waking everyone else up on the ward each time with the awful noise as the bed electronically moves. Thankfully I hear at least two of the others in the ward snoring, including the woman next to me, and so don't worry as much. Eventually, at about 2am, I am vaguely sleepy and comfy enough to manage to get some sleep while still listening to my iPod.

I jolt awake about half an hour later with a flashing alarm going off in the room and an instantaneous dream that this is my operation bell! The alarm is on the ceiling at the end of my bed, above the main doors, and flashing a red light and ringing full volume. I am just laying here not knowing what the ringing is for, wondering if someone is dying and this is the crash bell, and feeling physically sick and shaky as I have been woken too fast and have no idea what it was for. The alarm stops, no one comes into say there is a problem, or that it is not one that we are supposed to be concerned with. I manage to walk to the loo and cannot see any nurses anywhere to ask, and whilst I go back to my bed and iPod I have no chance of getting back to sleep- I'm far too shaky. So just try and relax as much as I can while listening to various meditations. It's not really working as the 'operation alarm bell' keeps ringing in my head, like some nightmare that's real. The snoring starts back up again but I just lie there, frozen to the sanctuary of my bed.

I get given more drugs in the morning (I think I am still on steroids) but get told I am not allowed any more than a few mouthfuls of water with them, and am impressed with myself that I manage to swallow them all with some water left.

18th May 07.36. Text to Dave.

> *"You awake yet? I've been up 2 hours, but shattered as kept waking up with alarms etc and now think I'm drugged! As feel groggy ☹ want a hug (was calm before the meds!) xx "*

(His reply- Are you ok?)

> *" …. No I'm as stressed as fuck*
> *I don't want it done but know I have no choice*
> *I want someone to hold me."*

Dave gets there early (it seems the visiting hours are mostly ignored in neurosurgery - I guess they know how much people are needed when their loved ones are having major operations) and comes and sits with me while I get given my hospital gown for surgery and lovely knee high anti DVT socks- with the non-slip ones for over the top! I was going to get Dave to help me have a shower, but I cannot get my energy up to do so and am shaking too much, so I just wash, brush my teeth, tie my hair up again in a high ponytail- so they can access the back of my head easier, and change into the gown in the bathroom instead.

Both the surgeons come round briefly, Timothy Jones tells me that he checked it was not full moon today, and jokes that there must be something odd in it as he married on a blue moon! I say yes I am ok with today, it's not full moon until the weekend. I'm scared, totally terrified, but ok.

Watching the clock hands turn is just awful… each minute seems like hours. I just feel sick to the core and wondering if this is it. What will happen during the operation? Will I survive? And if I do, what will I feel and be like afterwards. I am just numb with fear. I don't want to think about it, but can think of nothing else. The older women in the ward tell me I will be fine, remind me that they are very much older and have recovered well and that I am healthy and fit, so my operation will be fine. I wish I felt their positivity.

Eventually the nurses tell me they will take me down to surgery in a while. Do I want to be taken down in the wheelchair or bed? Neither really...do I have to? How far is it? Can't I just walk? So a few minutes later I walk myself down the corridor to theatre with Dave holding me up and a nurse walking alongside. Outside the door I give him a hug, tell him I love him, cry a bit more and walk in.

It's so clinical and scary in here, all white and super sterilised. It reminds me of the platform in Kings Cross in the Harry Potter films when Harry dies and meets Dumbledore. I guess having constant dizziness and blurry eyes doesn't help much. It has that horrid smell of hospitals magnified several times - the one that in my mind covers up blood and death. Oh I don't like this... I have to lay down on the table and I tell them I am terrified, the guy is really kind and talking to me, trying to reassure me and answer my questions about what they are doing and why. I am constantly talking and asking questions to try and reduce my insane fear. He attaches the heart rate monitor and I start to freak as I listen to the sound of it. As I listen, I can hear my heart beat going faster and faster, and the more I hear it going faster - the more I panic. Then the machine starts beeping and it goes even faster. Am I ever going to survive this? Thankfully the anaesthetist comes in and turns the machine sounds off. Every so often it still beeps, but I can feel my heart rate gradually slowing down.

I cannot stop shivering, I am literally jolting as I am so cold and scared and so she puts a 'blanket' like a huge inflatable duvet over me and keeps filling it with hot air. I finally feel warmer and stop shaking so violently. Another nurse comes in and talks to me, she says she understands how awful it is to be having this done and tells me that she knows how safe most operations are now, but when she had to have surgery recently - the first time since she had children - she said everything took on a whole new meaning, and understood my fear. She just sat, listened and held my hand for a while. I am so grateful she is there. She also told me that if she ever needed brain surgery she would choose my surgeon - he has a great reputation and is really skilled, and she would trust him. Trust. I am back to trusting again. They start telling me there are going to put one cannula in my hand and do the rest once I am unconscious, so are here fiddling with my small, and cold, veins.

At this point I start silently mouthing, or maybe I was quietly talking? Telling the Angels I need them with me now. I need them to hold me, to protect me, to keep me safe throughout my operation... to help, support and protect the surgeon and others in the room ... as I feel the coldness going inside me and drift off...

Chapter 15 - Angels Next to Me

The next thing I remember is hearing Dave's voice, telling me "You've done it, Jo" and something jolted inside me enough to realise my bed was being moved - I assume to a ward after the operation. I am realising that I'm still alive. I made it. I didn't bleed to death during the operation. And I drift back off to sleep...

Then I realise a bit more, that they have allowed Dave, my Mum and Adam to see me. But I cannot say anything, I can't even really open my eyes properly. I mumble something about I will squeeze their hand when I mean yes. I don't think they understood. I just wanted to lean over and hug them all, but I couldn't. Then I heard someone say she needs to rest for a while, but what seems like 30 seconds later they are at the side of my bed. I still can't talk, and I don't understand why, until the nurse tells me the anaesthetic dries up your mouth and do I want a drink? I take a sip of water through a straw and I can move my mouth. Vaguely speak- for what seems like 5 seconds until I need another sip, and another.

I keep asking what the lump is in my neck as it feels so huge and when I am laying on it, it hurts, but I cannot avoid laying on it as it is so big. I get told that my hair is knotted under there and the lump is that. I cannot feel it myself as I can't yet get my arms up, but I am still not sure why my neck (going into my right shoulder) would be lumpy? After all they operated on my head. It doesn't feel like hair, not unless I have anaesthetic numbing the area too much still and so everything feels wrong. I know Dave and my mum tried to help me get the pillows straight and comfortable. The cuddly rabbit was brilliant as I could just prop up a small part of the left hand side of my head, so I felt even - with the lump on one side, rabbit on the other.

My family were with me for what seemed a very short while until the nurses then said they need to go home and leave me to rest. Dave gives me my iPod and as I tell him puts one earphone in my ear, turns the music on and leaves the iPod near my hand on the bed and leaves my phone on the table. I ask him for my homeopathy kit - I can see it on the table. He tells me I am not allowed to have anything yet and so he will bring it back later. I am too spaced out to argue or even really understand. Before the operation I had asked him after the surgery to put (if nothing else) Arnica in my water, so I just let it go.

I am still so thirsty and my mouth gets stuck together, so I agree with Sandra my nurse that each time I need water I will raise my hand as I couldn't talk or call her when my mouth was stuck- every time she looked at me, or my arm went up, I think she bought me a sip of water. She was brilliant.

While I was still in that land of in between, each time I shut my eyes I could see shadows of what I thought were the nurses on my right side, then it gradually dawned on me that there were no nurses there. Not even one, as when the real nurses did come over they were at the end of my bed or standing in a different position even to what 'an impression' would be such as if you looked at a red light and saw a blue shadow in that spot after. Yet there were clearly 3 of them, 3 separate shadows watching over me. Nor was there a 'doctor figure' at the other side of the room, near the sink, who was oddly tall and just watching me, arms folded...

Suddenly (as I was again asking the Angels to heal me) I get it... that I am being protected by three Angel nurses on my right and the bright figure at the other side of the room was either an Angel surgeon or Archangel...whatever, he had a massively bright light behind his tall figured shadow and a very calming presence- just knowing he was watching me was powerful and healing.

The four figures stayed with me every time I shut my eyes all that night - even after I was able to speak to the nurse more and answer her questions as to my name and where I was. At this time, although I felt safe and protected, I was sure something had gone 'wrong' - I had heard something being said that I thought was implying that I was 'ok now'- and I could also see a bloody tube in my left hand, so I assume this is my blood transfusion drip? Several hours later I get the energy to ask Sandra (my nurse for the night) "So what went wrong?"

She replied slightly confused "Nothing did. Although the operation took longer than planned" (I think what I misunderstood as going wrong when still half out of it) "but you are doing great and you haven't yet needed any blood!"

I ask incredulously "What not even in theatre?" and she answers "No, none" and tells me she is just talking the last sample of my blood to check my levels, but if it is still ok I wouldn't need a transfusion. The bloody tube was where they were checking my blood from - not putting it in me! It was like someone had just told me I'd won a million pounds...I cried tears of relief and was thanking Angels so much for helping me. I had done this! Survived my hell, and I was ok and hadn't even had to have the blood transfusion I was dreading! It was about after I felt this joy that the Angel shadows disappeared.

Still most of the night it seemed all I could hear was the bloke opposite (I could just hear a male voice) having a wee into a bottle or his monitor machine going off and bleeping. It seemed every time I managed to vaguely sleep I was woken with this bleeping - like it was an alarm clock shocking you back into reality! Thankfully I managed to see the machine (but not him) and so could see it was his monitor with red lights flashing (and then I knew it was not mine- which helped me calm my panic!) The other woman on the ward was diabetic and was having to have her insulin checked every so often, then she felt sick … so I just stay there, still awake even with my iPod on and trying, but failing, to sleep. Mostly I only have an earphone in one ear, but at times I use them both, when I need to try and block out more noises and don't need to talk to anyone. I am trying to visualise and feel my hug from Roan - we both had our cuddly rabbit toy with us to hug, our substitutes for now.

Somewhere in the night I also start holding my fingers together to see if it feels like I can write or draw anything small with a pen, writing my name invisibly on the bed. Feeling an overwhelming sense that I have to do 'something positive' with my life now. This is my second chance. Knowing somehow I need to help others- and that I can, if I can just figure out what it might be.

In the morning, when the nurses pulled the curtains back, I think the guy in the bed opposite looked at me very weirdly - probably as I had been saying thank you 'to myself' half the night! I'd realised from his talking to the nurses that this was his second operation on his brain tumours, and I assumed he obviously had something medical that needed the nurses to check him, due to the constant bleeps, so I just tried to smile hello. However, not long after breakfast was offered (which he didn't want) he then unhooked himself off all the machines, had someone bring him in a stinky fat filled burger, ate it and then said he was going downstairs for some 'air'! All night I had been awake - a large proportion because of his machines bleeping, and yet he just unplugs himself and walks out in the morning- assumedly for a cigarette - I could scream!

I mention to Sandra, how much this machine bleeping had disturbed me all night and now he has just walked out for air! She tells me I should have said as she could have turned the sound down. I ask her does the hospital do a guide for patients with sensory issues, as it would be really helpful to know in advance what all the noises are, and she says no. We agree they need one.

I try and sit up a little and my head feels like I am on a spinning fairground ride, so I have to lie back down again- almost as low as I was previously and then slowly manage to sit up a tiny bit at a time without my dizziness going off on an insane scale. I even eat a few rather disgusting rice pops and soya milk (this was the only thing that there was available that was wheat and dairy free) without dropping any on myself- either that or I couldn't see that I did! I eat them slowly, mainly as I don't want to feel sick from eating too much on an empty stomach that's been recently anaesthetised; but also it still feels like I am in a drug like dream state with only half of me responding, the rest is still numb and dizzy. But I know I just have to do the actions anyway, re connect my brain.

After eating I manage to pick up my mobile phone and to play a game of solitaire. I need to see if my brain, hands and eyes still function alright. Yes! I complete it in just over 3 minutes, about my normal slow speed, but I could do it fine! I could think what I needed to do and touch the screen ok- even if I felt a little nauseous looking at phone for that time. So I put it down afterwards, but happy that at least some of me still works.

The new nurses came on duty and as I had started moving around a tiny bit more, I started hurting - my lower neck felt like I had a brick inside it. I asked one of the nurses for my Arnica tablets (as I know they reduce bruising and have felt the amazing pain relief from taking them many a time) and when I realise they are not here, ask does the hospital have any? She checked and said they could not give them from the hospital as they didn't have any in the chemist there. But as the nurse also couldn't use painkillers very well and used Arnica too - she understood how I felt and that they worked. But then another (main) nurse heard and said I would not be allowed Arnica anyway.

"What the fuck?" Cue a mini pain filled rant to a doctor and nurse roughly implying that doctors cannot say that homeopathy tablets are 'sugar pills' and also not let me use them as they interfere with the drugs... it doesn't make sense! Eventually I am asked by the doctor "Is it homeopathic arnica, or herbal arnica you want to take?" and they agree I could use homeopathic remedies, but not take herbal products as they might interfere with the drugs I had been given. That's fine...I just want my homeopathy kit. Now, please.

The 'arnica using nurse' then phoned Dave to tell him to bring my kit, on the first call he said he was not able to leave yet and would be there for visiting hours (that afternoon!) I just cried and begged her to call him again - and that I needed them NOW. I couldn't remember my Mum's phone numbers, the nurse could not find my next of kin details I had given the hospital (that should be on their system with my Mum's numbers on.) So on the second phone call, with me all but screaming at him in the background as the nurse called, Dave agreed to leave soon!

At some point before Dave arrives the surgeon comes round with all the students in tow (talking lots of medical stuff that I didn't really want to hear) saying he was happy the operation went well, that he was totally sure it a hemangioblastoma (but they still have to send it off to be tested) and he was pleased with how I was doing. Reminded me that I would be feeling dizzy for a while and it would probably be far worse than before the operation - you aren't kidding! Also that due to my funny head shape and a sticking out part in the centre of my head, they cut my head in an S shape instead to the right side. Typical- even my skull isn't normal!

Then I went to move my hair back off my face and touched near my drain tube at the top of my head. So I get told that this is now the third time he has seen me do this - apparently I touched my head straight after the operation and again when he saw me sometime after (which means I have probably touched it several times more.) So the tube needs removing ASAP. They will clip it now and if all is ok by the evening, they will remove it then. As after all "You have done so well with the operation it's not much point you dying of meningitis now is it?"

But I 'have' touched it. I know I have. Even he has seen it three times! It's a gut reaction of a mix of long hair that isn't tied up getting in the way, my dizzy vision and blurriness that make me want to push, my non-existent, glasses up on my head to see properly (I had my eyes lazered several years ago- but wore glasses that slipped down when half asleep for 20 years before that); as well as wanting to just hold my head still to help keep my vision straight and stop everything spinning. Not to mention that my whole head feels numb - and you want to touch numbness to find some type of feeling. Plus I have no mental image of where the tube is in my head and where not to touch. I can't see where it is, the only way to know would be to see it in a mirror or feel it!

But now I am worried, no, make that scared senseless, over what germs I could have put directly into my brain! Couldn't they have put a dressing on it, or sterile gloves on me and changed them frequently … or something… as I know I have touched my head several times. Oh bloody hell! I will try and not touch it anymore… but know I will.

Dave arrives and I tell him to not let me touch my head then grab my homeopathy from him, I half spill my arnica tablets all over the bed as I can't see them properly, nor tell if it's just one I have got, or even look down much. But the pain relief from the arnica was at least as good as the pain killers I had been given from hospital and it feels like the neck swelling is subsiding, I have more movement and it's hurting far less.

19th May 11.49. Dave kindly takes a picture of me as he is amazed I am sitting up, eaten and have played a game on my phone.

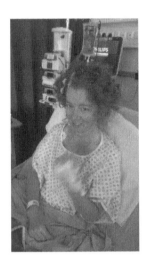

19th May, 11.51. I send a text to Nicola. It makes me feel a little nauseous looking at the screen, but I can type ok.

"It's me! And done! Been asking Angels all yest"

(Reply- OMG... how are you?? Did you have transfusion -I was fully intending that you would not ☺)

"OK ish! Getting there! and no I didn't have one ♥ ♥

Am sure I had angel nurse figures by my bed when I came round ... ❤"

The nurses tell me I will be moving back to the main ward as soon as they have a bed there, which I am amazingly happy about. Although also a little confused as I was told I would be in special care for a couple of days. The woman who I spoke to online who had the same operation also said she was in the high dependency care for several days and was quite 'out of it', as was another person I knew who had brain surgery.

I get the catheter removed, moved out of special care as my bed and I get pushed back to the ward I was in before; then told to try and get some sleep as Dave goes off to get lunch.

Chapter 16 - My Head is Spinning

14.10. Texts to Dave.

> *"Can you get me a 'sport top' water bottle when you come
> back please x
> PS. I think typing is easier!!!!*
>
> *I'm not sleeping- do you want to come back? Everyone else's
> visitors are here...."*

It is odd, as I have had brain surgery ending less than 24 hours ago, my head is totally spinning just like I have severe flu, but even writing a text is somehow easier already. I can co-ordinate where my fingers touch the screen better and so make less mistakes typing. Although the nausea from looking at a small bright screen when everything is spinning makes it a little hard, as if I concentrate on anything for too long I feel sick. That same feeling of travel sickness, when any time you get an unexpected movement your stomach seems to turn upside down, and well my vision is giving me lots of unexpected movements! I can't read or do anything intense for more than a minute at a time and the closer I am looking at something, the harder it is.

When Dave returns I add my Arnica and Hypericum tablets to the water bottle, so I have one drink to sip regularly to help with pain, and another drink for when I need water. I feel it's so much harder to do some things due to the dizziness and I don't feel I can see things properly, but I am coordinated enough to tip out a tablet and take a drink when I need to- even if the straw is still easier than drinking from a glass when laying slightly upright in bed.

I have to walk to the toilet. I have my (now clipped) head drain still connected to a wheeled stand, so I get Dave to check the drip wire is not tangled on anything, as I still can't turn much at all, then get up extremely slowly. First I twist round to put my feet off the side of the bed, then get Dave to put on the non-slip socks, and manage to stand up by myself while holding on to the stand for a bit of support, then wheel myself outside to the loo with Dave holding my other arm and a nurse in tow. I am thankful my bed is by the door and the toilet almost opposite as I am insanely dizzy and don't have much energy to walk. The nurse asks if I want anyone to come in the toilet with me. "Um, no thanks. I won't lock the door and will call if I need you." I somehow manage the now complicated act of having a wee and now understand why they have full length mirrors on the wall opposite the toilet in the neurosurgery ward. They are useful when you cannot move your head to look down! Having to flush the loo, pull my clothes together, press the soap dispenser, wash my hands and dry them suddenly now seems like a hard task. I feel I am double checking if I am doing things ok and in the right order as part of me has forgotten. Once again I feel like it is a drunken dream. I ask Dave to check I am decent as I walk out, as I cannot look behind me at all yet.

When the consultants come round to check on me I ask why my neck feels so swollen and sore, as it seems as though I have had a small brick surgically attached to my neck just under my skin. They tell me it's as they had to cut through my neck muscles to get to my skull. Oh! I didn't realise that, but now the pain makes more sense and that I haven't got something odd going on in my neck that no one has picked up on!

19th May 15.15. Dave kindly takes more pictures of me.

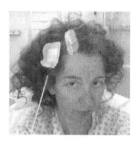

19th May 15.53

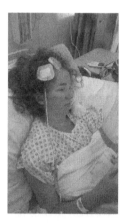

I walk to the toilet again, this time I manage to walk myself back and it wasn't too horrendous, but I don't feel like drinking too much water and needing this trip too often. It's really hard trusting that you won't faint or fall over from the dizziness, and it still seems really hard to even remember what order you do even the simple acts of flushing the loo and washing your hands. Everything seems just a little unreal and fluffy round the edges. I guess a nice mixture of getting anaesthetic out my system, drugs and the fact someone was inside my skull yesterday.

A bit later when Dave has gone for a break, I take pictures of myself on my phone - so I know where my head drain is (and where not to touch!) I still can't yet see it properly in the bathroom mirror as I cannot stand upright and still long enough nor see it that clearly with the spinning and blurry vision. It's not a pretty photo. I look like a mad woman with my hair glued in a total sticking up mess and a slightly puffy face! Not that I really care - glamour isn't high on my list of concerns right now, but I look like I had a really rough night last night!

Some point that afternoon the consultants see me going on another trip to the loo and are impressed I am already up walking, so they wait in the ward and ask me to walk a little up the centre of the room once I am done. I manage to put one heel next to the toe on the other foot!! It touched and I didn't fall over. Blimey! - I haven't done this for months! Months! Yet I can do it less than 24 hours after the operation! Plus, despite the insane dizziness, I feel I am already walking in a straighter line than before the operation, somehow my body is regaining its balance. Wow! I'm impressed! As are they.

I manage to eat dinner- some awful tasting processed chicken curry and rice, but I could physically manage to eat it. The hot temperature of the food feels it is burning my throat (which was feeling very sore after the operation, and is seemingly worse today) but also actually helping it. I just about manage to get the food into my mouth, despite the coordination issues, and swallow it. I feel a bit like I am just trying to shovel it in, but not finding my mouth easily so who cares where it goes, but I think it felt worse than reality and I didn't make too much of a mess. Again due to the sore throat and swollen feeling in my neck I feel I cannot swallow fully, so just have to keep eating small mouthfuls and drinking lots of water.

Later that evening Mum arrives with Zach - just as one of the doctors turns up to remove my brain fluid drainage tube. I tell Zach he is going back outside. Even if he wanted to watch, I don't want him to see this, I know I have the risk of having a fit, and that is not something I wish him to see, so he and Mum leave the room. At this point I am very thankful I cannot see the top of my head! Dave stays and I lean my head on him, shutting my eyes and attempting to relax, while they give me a local anaesthetic and slowly pull out the drainage tube. It feels like a long piece of string coming out of my skull. Dave asks can he video it, or take a photo ("NO!") then graphically tells me how long the tube is, and how much it stretches, all whilst the doctor is removing it. But the tube is out of me already, seemingly without much fluid in it, when I was told it would be in for 3 days plus while it drained. They put a stitch in my head afterwards and leave me with my family. We chat for a little while then Zach, Mum and Dave all go home.

I try and take some photos of the top of my head where the drainage tube cuts are. I know I had two areas with plasters on them, and the tube has now gone and is stitched up, so I assume I can look closer without such an infection risk. (Not that I would dare touch it still!) I try and take some selfies of my head. I take loads in the attempt to get a picture I can see. I have no idea how far away to hold the phone or what angle to take them, and am not even totally sure where the scars are. So have to delete a load of blurry pictures, but after several minutes I have a couple that clearly show I have staples in my head and a bald patch! I thought I was just getting a drainage hole.

19.18

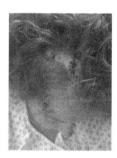

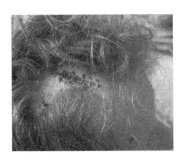

I am sitting looking at my photos of the surgery done on me... and I suddenly don't get why I am in here, in hospital, in a brain surgery ward, where brain tumours are removed! Why me? What did I do to cause this? I don't drink, I don't smoke, I don't eat junk- heck, I don't even eat gluten, I try and eat organic and avoid pesticides, I don't use fluoride, I avoid using mobile phones, Wi-Fi and other EMF's and I try and avoid toxins in my skincare and household products. Yet I have just had a brain tumour removed! A large fucking BRAIN tumour. This is like some odd dream...

19.57. Text to A

> *"Stressful last night and this morning as neck really bruised and sore from cutting the muscles, but slowly getting better and seeing and dizziness better than earlier too.*
> *It just feels really wrong and not real tho...and why???*
> *But some in here have cancerous tumours in front of brain- really not nice to see or hear* ☹
> *Problem is when it was only 24 hrs after op I was getting frustrated as I wasn't better! And I have to be in 5 days plus ...*
>
> *And yes ... time... I know it will take a while, but I still would like the magic wand* ☺
> *Surgeon seems impressed with himself tho! Not that I mind, but I think it's good on his CV* ☺*"*

At some point in the evening I walk back in from another toilet trip (I am now walking alone - I just make sure nurses know where I am before I go into the toilet) and ask the woman in the opposite bed how old 'her baby' was? (She had been talking to someone on an online video messenger and calling them her baby earlier) ... she tells me her baby she was speaking to is a dog, and her son is 26! I mutter something about him missing her while I have a really sickening sense of déjà vu that I have witnessed this exact scene before- of me speaking to someone in a hospital bed about their baby and it being a dog. Hmmm... was I always going to have this operation no matter what I did? Did this scene have to happen? Is that why I dreamt this before? Whatever the reason, I feel a bit calmer that I did have to have this operation. That it was part of my soul's journey and all would now be OK.

At medicine round I get given the steroids and paracetamol and also told I need a heparin injection to stop blood clots, I still have the anti-DVT socks on but apparently I need the heparin too. I get told I can have it in my stomach or arm. I ask which one works best and hurts less, and get told that in the stomach I will not feel it as they can inject into fatty areas, whereas sometimes it can make your arm ache.

I must have odd pain threshold as I can feel the coldness of the injection hitting my belly, and within a short while it feels sore. Empty and sore. I want to rub it, but get told I shouldn't - due to the fact its heparin. So gradually I feel more and more nauseous and my belly is increasingly painful. Not agony just a raw sore pain where I cannot touch it. My belly then feels a strange sense of numbness, that where I touch somehow isn't being felt by my pain sensors, it feels like I have a layer of something over my skin where I can't quite get the correct sensations from even a gentle touch.

The nurses seem to think that I cannot be nauseous and have pain from the heparin but it's either that, the paracetamol (which I know can easily happen with me) or the anaesthetic coming out... or just a mix of all three! I take some more homeopathy advised for after anaesthetic and get more wind and pains, and the nausea starts to subside.

20.52. Text to Dave.

> *"Medicine round now!!* ☹
> *And had a fucking injection for stopping blood clots* ☹ *but no choice yet again... This is so not me....but have to let go and trust them....*
> *I think that's my message - to let go of fear...*☹ *"*

("Be brave")

> *"I know...but it's so fucking hard* ☹
> *And now my tummy is sore (from injection) and I cannot even rub it..."*

As the night wears on, my neck pain seems to increase, the lump at the back feels like a brick inside me still which means I cannot get comfortable leaning on it at all, and there is an odd feeling at the front of my neck where the swelling seems to be affecting me. It almost feels like my windpipe is swelling up, but I can breathe ok. My right ear feels weirdly blocked and clicky. Everything is sore. I want to put my head on a pillow and sleep - after all I am totally exhausted - but I cannot, as whatever I try I cannot get comfortable for more than a few seconds. I have tried with the back of the bed upright as well as down flat and every angle in between, even tried putting the feet of the bed up to prop me up and stop me slipping down, with pillows at the side of my head, under the back of my head, I try to lie on my side, even roll round and lie on my front at various angles. Yet whatever I try is only comfortable for a minute or so maximum before the agony starts to hit. I cannot move my head much without it and my neck hurting, and I cannot turn to look at and arrange pillows or anything well, so much of it is done by feeling alone, so even moving from one position to another is hard. I am in agony, but it hurts to move, my neck hurts so much, so each time I try and turn I am gritting my teeth and silently (or not so silently) saying "Oh fuck!"

My head, rather disgustingly, feels like it has started clicking inside - similar to when your ears pop, but inside my head at the top and back of my skull. It's very odd to listen to and accept it's normal. My head feels achy - nowhere near as bad as it has been, but still aching none the less- and so I try and put my hand on my tailbone and bring the cerebrospinal fluid and pain down there. (I have felt the huge relief of a craniosacral therapist taking away my headaches - before I knew I had a brain tumour- by doing this) Happily I can feel the pain and clicking in my head reducing and my tailbone and hand pounding instead. Unfortunately, due to the fact I cannot get comfortable, I cannot hold my hand on my tailbone for long at a time, before I have to move position again. But it is working, it is so helping me.

Then somewhere in this discomfort, an ambulance crew brings a woman from another hospital into the empty bed in the ward. Whom every few minutes for the rest of the night keeps saying, almost shouting, really slowly and clearly like she is talking to a hard of hearing person, things such as "Can - I - have - a - bed - pan - pl-ease", "Nurse - I – need - a - bed -pan...now" … over and over. Even though some of the time when she was saying it the nurses had a bed pan with her or had just removed it. It is exhausting. Of course I feel sorry for her as she seemingly has been admitted from another hospital due to problems, isn't understanding what she is saying or doing, and (of course) she is on the brain tumour ward. I want to know why she is so 'out of it', what the problem is. Have a reason why this won't be me. Feel sick at the thought this could be me. Yet - I can't help, I cannot do a single thing to help. Although I really need to sleep and this is just another distraction to stop me doing so, and stress me further.

The nurses get me an ice pack to put on my neck to hopefully reduce the swelling, but it seems it is too solid to help as only a small area is being cooled and not at all comfortable to lie on. The nurses then, on my suggestion (I have four kids after all!), try a fan with a wet cloth wrapped around my neck... it seems to reduce the swelling and the tightness in my neck and the fresh air helps to cool the hot room down. Plus I have the added benefit that the fan makes a loud noise as it moves- which helps drown out more of the other sounds in the room I am trying to blank out.

20th May 00.51. Text to Dave.

> "No chance of sleep – neck feels insane ☹ this is really hard... we are really treating ourselves to something when this is over..."

And while I am my own state of struggle, I have the poor elderly woman in the bed next to me (the one that was rolling her arms in her sleep when I first was in this ward before the operation) groaning and writhing in pain all night - her machines keep bleeping, the nurses are constantly having to attend to her, something is obviously a problem, although I am trying to avoid hearing what. My music progresses from quiet relaxation music, to Muse, and in the end some loud Foo Fighters and Kasabian, and it is still not drowning out what is happening next to me. I cannot listen to her, I feel I absorb all the negative and fear. My empathy and anxiety levels are going through the roof, I feel it's me they are treating, not her. I cannot listen to it...I need to heal me.

The nurses seem to be doing all sorts of things to this woman next to me. I am hearing too much, even though my music is on as loud as I can manage. I am asking myself how loud should you have earphones on after a brain operation? Would this increase the risk of a fit? It seems many here have had one after their operation. The iPod is on at least ¾ of the maximum volume, yet it seems all I can hear is her groaning, with bleeps and buzzers going off everywhere. I literally cannot cope with this, so at some point while they are sorting her out I get out of bed and go and sit at the nurse's station outside. Anywhere but in that damn room. I am crying with exhaustion and start chatting to the only person there, a second year student nurse who has only been on this ward a few days. I ask her how she copes, how does she manage with the constant bleeps, buzzers and bells? She tells me that she is still getting used to it, it is much noisier here than on the previous ward she worked on. But she understands me, she says "I can see why you cannot sleep and how you can easily panic with each bleep." She tells me she gets taught what alarms are 'more serious' and which are 'routine monitoring', and agrees that it would be helpful if patients could also be told this. We decide the only option left to help me reduce the pain and possibly manage to sleep is taking another dose of morphine - great!

I sit at the nurses station, ear bashing this lovely student nurse (the same age as my eldest son) for about an hour, spewing out all my fears, confusion and anger on her while she amazingly and patiently listens; until I feel I will fall asleep sitting upright on the chair next to her. The morphine seems to have kicked in and I cannot manage any more. I go back to my bed with my music back on as loud as possible, put my hand on my tailbone as I manage to fall asleep for a couple of hours even with all the pain and distractions...

Chapter 17 - Get Me Out of Here

20th May 06.26. Text to Dave

> *"God that was a bad night!!! Had woman next to me being treated and groaning for ages...so I am freaking even listening to IPod – had to go outside in the end and cry at nurses. Swear heparin injection had made me feel nauseous- or paracetamol? My guts just keep glugging. Can move neck again tho. And I finally fell asleep...*
> *So tired tho still...I want a hug*
> *And don't bring Roan today... "*

> *"And if you can, can you buy a new comb with different width teeth- and some soft hair bands- I look like a witch ☹"*

> *"I want you here...as I know I can fall asleep again then ...*
> ❤ *"*

("Try to go to sleep and I will pop up later")

> *"I want to...but it's so hard! I had another morphine last night and suddenly clonked for a while after- woke up thinking 'fucking hell, did I sleep?'*
> *I want someone to reassure me what I am feeling again...I think stuff is pulling together on head.*
> *Trying to trust its reconnecting as it needs to... x"*

(Do you have dreams?)

"No dreams as not asleep. Am feeling neck is better (and MUCH less swollen than last night!) but have tingle on and off in head- around where tumour was, I guess its gotta grow back neuron connections...
Clicking head noise doesn't feel as bad atm- but have had to have music on all night...
I know I am stressed tho...and just want to be away from the bleeps and rushing around...its freaking me too much ☹*"*

(Jo the more relaxed you are, the better your recovery. Looking at some people in your ward, looks like your recovery is very good so far ☺
Please try and relax, is there anything I can bring you later than may help relax you?)

"Camomile tea and mint tea. A book on brain tumours and what sensations you may get after ... ☺*"*

(I will bring the tea, not the book)

"And a hug...I need a hug...about a years worth x
I'm so sorry...I never wanted to do this to you and kids....
It's just not real..."

I feel like shite, I'm aching and sore. Exhausted. Stressed as anything. Still worried that I might have got an infection before they took my tube out. Worried I may have a fit. Want to know will everything really be ok. Don't really know if the sensations in my head are ok or not. Can't stand being alone. Can't stand listening to all these bleeps, lights, buzzers and calls. Yet I somehow acknowledge that this is the lowest part and so I take another few selfies to remind myself what hell feels like and how it can only get better.

6.58am

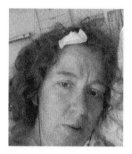

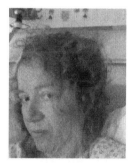

I send a text back to A (who asked me how my night was)

> *"I had relaxing music on for hours! Have gone through Foo Fighters and Kasabian when needed the noise... now on Muse! I can tap my feet to that and get some chill, even when I want to cry!*
> *I so want to go home and cuddle my babies ...*
> *Doesn't help when I panic I know as it makes it worse...it just feels so bloody slow...*
> *But it's out...its gone..."*

I also seem to have this on/off buzzy feeling in my head - like the area the tumour was in is now vibrating. Thankfully one of the student consultants tells me "does it feel like a bee is buzzing inside?" and tells me that sensation seems to be common after surgery. Also that the clicking noise inside, pain and rest of it is normal. It is so reassuring to hear that the sensations are to be expected. I am also feeling somewhat better as the neck pain and swollen feeling has reduced and so I refuse the morning dose of paracetamol as I really can do without the nausea that comes with it. I am instead still swigging my (freshly topped up) water bottle of homeopathic remedies.

Sometime in the morning they realise the woman in the bed next to me has a blood clot and so it is panic stations as they get people in to diagnose and then plan to move her off to another part of the hospital... but I cannot listen to any of it. I am going insane as I think she is about to die in the bed next to me. I don't know what to do. I want to run away from here as I cannot take it anymore.

09:43. Text to Dave

> "When you come in PLEASE can you get it into the nurses that I am freaking with this woman next to me...I feel I am on constant adrenaline panic mode and so cannot heal or sleep.
> When I try and sleep I keep having nightmares they are talking about me not her. I am exhausted from all the bleeps etc...or would they listen if you phoned...I am on iPod on full volume but cannot turn it down as I just cannot hear noise without feeling worse...
> It's like living in A&E...horrendous"

After sending this text I realise I have to do something now and go outside to the nurses and literally cry at them saying I have to be moved away from this ward. I cannot cope and it's affecting me badly. The nurse tells me that she can take me to the treatment room for a while - where it is quiet - and they will sort another bed as soon as they can. I grab my iPhone and go, I can't even manage to walk back into the ward and all the chaos to get my iPod and the music on it. The nurse walks me down to the room, shows me where the buzzer is, lets me sit down on the hard couch 'examining bed', gives me a pillow and leaves me there.

Text back to Dave- who has told me he is on his way to the hospital.

> *"I have now been moved to a treatment room for a while to calm…but just panicking!…*
> *It's just more than I can hack now…I'm shattered…*
> *Am calming down now….*
> *Slowly x"*

> *"Don't want to be by myself tho… as know how long they take to answer bells…"*

I only have my phone with me but I find some healing apps on it that I had previously started to download when I thought my operation was in a week's time. Although they are only the free introductions they have relaxation sounds which help me and then I find another part that has a calming meditation. It's only a few minutes long, but I play it over and over. I also ask the angels continuously to help calm and heal me and a few minutes' later feel a calming presence and see a violet healing light behind my closed eyes which starts to calm me. (Violet is the colour that I always see when I have a deep meditation treatment.) I want to fall asleep sitting here - although as I am in a room at the end of a corridor totally alone I decide it's not the best option.

> *"Am calm now x and really want to fall asleep where there are no constant noises..."*

Dave texts me back to say he has arrived, parked and is just walking into the hospital. I manage to get up and sit by the door of the treatment room until he arrives. When he gets inside I just sit and cry at him with the total exhaustion of it.

Chapter 18 - Mind Over Matter

After a while a therapist turns up to assess the swallowing /sore throat issues I am having. So of all the things that feel awful the staff think this is a problem?! She feels my throat and tests how I swallow and then gets me to eat a small amount of fruit while she again feels my throat, the banana is OK, but apple is harder and feels like it is stuck in my throat. She insists that it is not and that it is just the after effect of the tube down my throat for 5 hours during the operation.

I can't remember how long I sat in the treatment room, and I am not sure for how long I went back to the old ward for (minus the older woman next to me) but I think I ate lunch there with the curtains drawn around me while I tried to relax with Dave. I was too tired to really notice.

14:33 Text to Nicola. (Asking how long I would be staying in hospital)

> "Not sure how long, but was told 5 days was min before op. So Sunday? But possibly Monday as do they kick you out on Sunday? But I can feel it's starting to get better... my neck swelling is going down, no head ache (tho a bit odd and numb) and I can type this easier than before op...and I actually managed to walk with my feet in a straight line today! (drunk test!) Not perfect but better than I was in January!! ☺
> Going to move me to a quieter bed soon ☺"

I get told I now have a new room, so they move my bed to a smaller ward with lower dependency, further up the corridor. It can only fit four beds inside, but there are only two other people in here right now. One is an older woman who doesn't say why she is here, but tells me she was an ex- midwife and seems chatty and kind. The other is a woman about my age who says she also had a brain tumour removed, but went home, did too much, relapsed and now she is back in here- and tells me several times to take it easy when I go home and don't rush the healing. But this ward is so much quieter as even despite someone having their TV on loud it feels more normal, there are no bleeping machines, it seems cooler and lighter plus the women are able to talk ok. Maybe I can finally sleep later today and also tonight?

After a while a neuro-physiotherapist turns up to assess me. She starts with checking my balance, so I stand next to the bed while she tests me and if I can stand with my feet together, or with my eyes shut etc. Then she asks how well I can walk. This time I manage to walk a few steps with my heel to toe together!!! The next challenge is walking up and down the corridor looking to one side of the corridor wall while I am walking and then turning to look at the other side, the ceiling and the floor- again far better than before the operation as I can actually look to my side ... and ... I don't fall over! It is more than a little like a drunken dream of wobbliness, but still somehow better than it has been for the last few months. I feel I am spinning more, but I can control my body better, I even manage to stop when someone walks out of a doorway and not just crash into them. After this, she gets me to walk up the corridor to the staircase and to see if I can walk up and down the stairs. I can do it OK, even if I am feeling more than a little tired from the dizziness and the fact I have barely been able to move from my bed to the sofa for the past few weeks and that my energy levels are awful. But I will bloody do it, I will ignore the spinning and all the natural reflexes that tell me it's wrong to be walking, I know my head is supposed to spin after this operation, it is so much easier when you know there is a reason, so I put mind over matter and just get on with it.

The physiotherapist tells me that I did really well, she is impressed with my recovery so far. As they are not there over the weekend, the neuro-physiotherapy team will see me again on Monday to assess my going home routine, and then they will book me to come back and see them sometime after I go home. She tells me to keep stretching my neck over the weekend by looking as far as I can to the left and right, up and down.

I am sitting quietly, finally without my iPod playing in my ear, and Dave tells me he has a surprise for me in a while. Then a few minutes later my Mum walks in the door with Roan. He is obviously a little upset and scared by being at the hospital, but comes and sits on the bed next to me while we just hug and cry. He tells me he doesn't like my staples and Dave tries to cover my shaved bit of hair at the front by pulling another piece of hair over it, bald man style, and retying it (his attempt at a pony tail when my hair is glued up!) Roan tells me it is better as he cannot see the staples now and I look more normal.

While Roan and I are sitting on the bed hugging to make up for the last few days of not being able to see each other, Mr Jones walks in. He tells me, Dave and Mum that he is really happy with how I am healing and the physiotherapy results … and that … I can go home.

I ask incredulously "What? I can go home today? Really?"

He nods his head and smiles … and I just cry and squeeze Roan harder. Then I tearfully say "Dave has just thought 'oh shit', but your nurses will be happy!"
Mum says "Oh blimey, I'd better go home and tidy up and change your bed sheets". And I just cry a bit more, and ask Mr Jones if they are fed up with me in hospital.
"No, you have just reached all our discharge targets."

He gives us info on how and when to wash my hair - I can wash it gently tomorrow, although it may need lots of shampoo to remove the glue and it will take a couple of washes to go fully, and do so only by showering as I cannot lie in the bath. Plus I need the staples removed next Friday and they will give me the remover to do so at my local surgery as any nurse or doctor can do it.

He tells me it will take a few hours for them to discharge me with the medications and everything, but that I can go home as soon as they do.

I am then laughing at him that one day he will see me when I am not crying! As I just keep tearfully saying thank you.

Roan gets another huge cuddle and cries with me that I will be home with him again tonight. He and my Mum go home shortly after to go and tidy the house - not before the other kids receive a call to get the vacuum out and wash up. I sit on the bed and smile like an insane Cheshire cat.

A nurse takes the dressing off the back of my head before I go - Dave takes a photo as we realise the length of the scar and the amount of staples in my head. I realise it looks like I have a (bloody) zip in my head... and laugh that it's a shame it's not Halloween!

16.49

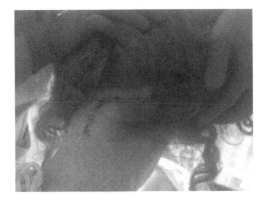

I feel totally shocked, I am grinning insanely - I am going home TODAY! Yet am simultaneously trying to work out if I can manage at home with no one to ask who knows about brain surgery, as I still have so many questions.

I sit on the bed and try and work out how to do what feels like everything at once. I get rid of the anti DVT socks and silly hospital gown and change into some leggings and a stretchy top - I brought a few clothes online once I knew I was needing an operation that I could pull up over my hips and so avoid them going over my head. Get Dave to tidy the worst of my hair up by tying it up again. Try and sort through my few bags and put my iPod, phone, charger and belongings into bags. It is insanely weird to do so, I still feel the world is spinning and I can't quite focus straight, but I am so ready to go home. I am talking stupidly excitedly fast and have found an extra burst of energy amidst the tiredness and lack of sleeping for the past week. Dave tells me to slow down and don't rush as we will still be ages, but I want to be ready as soon as they are. I want to go home. I want to go home and cuddle my baby.

I send a text to almost everyone on my phone contact list:

"Coming home today! *"*

Chapter 19 - 48 Hours After Surgery

While we are waiting to be discharged, the food trolley arrives. I have been advised as it may still be a while before the nurses get all my medicines from the pharmacy and the discharge papers that I should probably eat. However, despite me booking in at my pre op appointment as needing gluten free food and asking staff every time they bring the menu round, they have managed to use up all the gluten free meals! (And the only gluten free option on the menu to start with was a jacket potato- not exactly great for a main meal!) So I get the only thing vaguely edible on the trolley, which is a banana, to eat while I am waiting. Thankfully I am going home tonight! I can go back to organic food and avoid the waxed and polished, freakily snow white looking, apples and processed junk that they have here and aren't exactly health promoting.

Finally the nurses bring round my drugs... basically a load of painkillers along with two steroid tablets and a box of the tablets that need to be taken with them to reduce stomach symptoms. Why I get whole box of these when I only have 2 steroid tablets and only need to take one with each, and why I need senna tablets when I have already told the nurses I won't take senna, I have no idea. But the nurse tells me they are prescribed and so it is easier for me to take them home than her trying to return them to their pharmacy!

But I only need to take the steroids for another two days. 2 more days!! That is such brilliant news, as it will only be 7 days in total that I have needed to take them. I had been thinking that I would have to take medications, and possibly these steroids, for months. I don't have to even consider whether I need to continue taking them and 'be good' or argue as to why I don't want to... yippee! I can manage 2 more days!

I get told I need to have my staples removed in 7 days' time - on Friday next week - and get given the correct 'surgical tweezers' to remove them along with the instructions on the sterile bag. I'm again told that any nurse or G.P. will be able to remove them as they are no different to removing stitches, and they will all be able to do that. So now I have all my discharge papers and medicine... I can go home!

I leave the ward still smiling, laughing and crying at the same time. Dave has to hold my arm to steady me and we walk slowly arm in arm down the corridor. The same corridor I walked down to go into theatre, as the operating theatre is opposite the lift we need to use, the only seating near there is by the lift doors. Dave tells me how long he sat outside there, just looking at the theatre doors during my operation. Watching different heads being wheeled out and being taken to the wards, until he saw a redhead with her arms in the air, and knew it was me. While I cry even more.

He tells me that after I walked into the operating theatre that the nurse told him she has never had a patient walk themselves down to theatre before- and that I must have strength. Another load of tears roll down my cheeks. Really? Is walking to theatre strong? Walking seemed far more logical than being taken in a wheelchair or bed. But, I guess, I also needed to have 'some' control over this...

We go down in the lift and across near the main neurology block entrance. I then find a chair to sit down on while Dave goes to get the car from the car park so he can stop in the patient collection bay just outside.

I see a woman who was with me in the ward walking out of the small shop there with her husband. She comes over to ask me am I going already and tells me she is pleased for me. She was barely able to speak when I saw her before my operation, but is now able to walk around and talk, albeit carefully and slowly like she is having to pronounce the words very clearly. She tells me she cannot leave hospital yet, but tells me how much better she is than they expected as the doctors said she may not have been able to speak for a few months - due to where her tumour was. I tell her how much better she seems and it's good to hear her talking ok and she tells me she is happy with how she is doing, as does her husband. Then she tells me she still has to fully address the cancer, and when she leaves here will start further treatment. She is amazed I am leaving and wishes me good luck. I fully realise how lucky I am.

Dave arrives back inside the building, guides me into the front passenger seat of the car and we leave St George's. It's just past 6pm, almost exactly 48 hours from when I left theatre.

The drive back home is the oddest one ever... Tooting and Wimbledon look similar to what England does when you arrive back in the country after a holiday where the land you have been is much less green, or almost as a foreign city looks to a tourist when you see it for the first time. I just see it as different - more colourful and amazing somehow. Yet it is only 4 days ago I was being driven in the opposite direction and it seemed a shithole! I am looking at the date plaques on the houses, the sculpture of the brickwork and chimneys, imagining the houses as they were when they were built in the year on the plaques. I just don't care if it takes us 2 hours to get back - I am going home! I survived!! Every so often this realisation hits me again and I just cry. I did it. I fucking did it.

Each time a car pulls out in front of us, it just doesn't matter. They don't know what I have had done and maybe they had a shitty day at work? It is Friday afternoon in rush hour after all. They have their own issues in their lives and I don't care if they slow us up. I occasionally feel travel sick and need to shut my eyes, plus going over any road bumps is horrendous and jolts my head too much, which isn't helped as I cannot lean my head against the head rest or it feels painful and more numb again. I'm totally high on the fact I have left hospital - and after only 2 days.

I get back home, plonk myself on the sofa and eat some of the food a friend has kindly bought round- a lovely gluten free chocolate cake with icing. It all tastes a bit odd, sensations feel wrong and numbed and I still feel I cannot properly swallow. It reminds me of eating when you have just brushed your teeth and nothing tastes right as it is all mint flavoured, but its more than just the taste that is wrong, it feels wrong too. I ask someone to lightly cool some boiled water for me and add lots of raw manuka honey in it, which is amazingly soothing and healing on my throat.

I manage to post this brief message on Facebook with my laptop - this is as much as I can write before the nausea from typing while looking at a 'moving' screen hits.

> *"I'm back home - just 48 hrs after end of op!!! Thank you all for your love, healing and prayers they really worked amazingly!* ♥ ♥ ♥
> *Thank you x"*

Although almost as soon as I finish I go to bed. My mum managed to get lovely clean fresh sheets on the bed, so it feels superbly soft and comfy after the starchy stiffness of hospital beds. I need to just sit down and relax in my space for a while. I am totally exhausted from the lack of sleep of what has now been a full week of not sleeping at night with just a few instances of two hours solid sleep in that time (well, apart from the actual operation). And this is me after all - if I get less than 7 hours sleep I am a bleary eyed zombie who needs to sleep in the afternoon and I can normally quite happily spend ten hours or more in bed! I start to panic as I can feel the exhaustion setting in, that everyone has left me upstairs to rest, and I don't know what to expect from my head, as well as the enormity of everything that's happened in the last few months starts to hit home.

I start to ask Angels to hold me, listen to more meditation and try to get comfortable in my V-pillow with loads more pillows propping me up. Which is hard when you cannot lean on your scar- and it feels like your scar covers almost half the back of your head! I constantly have to lean on the left side of my head and know my neck is twisted in that direction as I have not been able to lay or even sit straight for months. I also seem to get a strange tightening or buzzing sensation if I lean on the wrong area of my head, on top of the constant feeling that I have a layer of papier-mâché stuck on my skull. It is totally numb in patches when I touch it, and feels very swollen and tender still. Despite all this I manage to doze off for about forty minutes, until the neck pain from laying with my head bent totally to one side wakes me back up again.

Each time I need the toilet I have to shout to let the family know where I am going - as I daren't lock the toilet door (and no one wants to see you on the loo!) but also as getting up and walking is still this awful drunken confusing dream. I feel like I am faking being normal, that am really barely unable to get out of bed or open my eyes. Yet somehow I do it anyway. By about 9pm I have had enough and just want to go sleep properly so we organise a bedside table for me by bringing a small table up from downstairs- somewhere to keep my glass of water, a phone, homeopathy, painkillers, something to eat (to minimise the nausea from pain killers) and my arnica cream. The arnica cream is amazing! It feels like something is giving my neck a cooling soothing massage each time I get Dave to apply it and I can almost feel the swelling subsiding.

Roan comes up looking exhausted and tearful and asks me for a cuddle, but when I lay him next to me I realise I can't have him leaning his weight onto my body even a tiny bit as it increases the pain in my head. I feel awful as I so want to cuddle him and know that he needs a hug too, but we manage with him lying next to me leaning on the outside of my pillows, with my arm on him. As awkward as it is, I think it helps calm the both of us down.

After a while I sleepily sense Roan gets out of bed saying good night, and the next thing I know is I wake up a bit later realising Dave is next to me. But from then, all night I keep waking with a disgusting chemically sterile plastic taste and sensation in my mouth and the feeling that someone is trying to insert a tube down my throat. I can almost feel the soreness in my throat and have the fear of something horrible happening. I tell Dave what I am dreaming and keep asking him to hold me so I feel safe. So I know he is here and that no one will be able to do that to me again while I am asleep.

I am so uncomfortable, I cannot lean anywhere on my right side of my head, or lay straight when I am on my back, and have to tip my neck to the left a lot of the time- often with the toy rabbit as support to balance out the feelings. Which works for a while, until I start to seize up again and so have to try another position. About midnight I suddenly declare I need a ginger tea and I need it now, I feel sick and this 'operation taste' is so strong in my throat I need something to take it away. So a bleary eyed Dave gets me a cup of cooled ginger tea and after a few mouthfuls I can finally get some relief from the nausea that has been there since the operation. At about 2am I actually manage to lie on my front with my face wedged over the side of a V pillow and just clonk out until 7am or so.

Chapter 20 - Trying to Heal

The next couple of days blur into a head spinning state of sleeping, attempting to watch TV, working out how to get to the loo and back, eating, and going back to bed by 9pm totally exhausted. I need 2 naps a day and literally feel I am beginning to stop functioning each time before I fall asleep. I was told I could wash my hair on Saturday, but I cannot manage to summon the energy to get in the bath. I feel far too drunk and my head is just far too sore and numb- it feels tight and I am aware of it at all times. If anyone touches it, it makes the numbness feel worse both as I realise I cannot feel a thing and it seems my muscles tighten and increase this horrid feeling. If it is touched or I lean on it the 'wrong' way, I feel like I am leaning on a metal plate that's digging in inside my head. When I wake or have been sitting in the same position too long I feel like I have slept with my neck bent and somehow cut the blood off so it feels tingly. Sometimes I just have to lie down on my left side and get all the sensations to subside a little.

Evening of 21st May. Mum comes round to babysit me (or provide me with food, drinks and company) while Dave and Zach are off playing a previously booked gig. One that was supposed to be before my operation and not the day after I come home. I ask Dave if he is too tired to go, but he says he needs the normality and could do with a break. All evening I don't manage to do much apart from walk from the sofa to the loo a couple of times, and then go to bed. When Dave comes back he seems to crash out as soon as his head hits the pillow, while I feel simultaneously wired (I am still taking these steroids) and exhausted at the same time, and too tired to sleep easily. I thought he was supposed to be keeping an eye on me, not the other way round.

Late on Sunday morning I get into the bath and Dave attempts to wash my hair with the shower, in the way we have been told to get rid of the glue, while I am sitting down in the warm water ... my hair is still knotty, covered in glue and my whole head feels numb. Sitting down I cannot manage to even hold my hands up for more than a few seconds to touch my head as the muscles start to ache. But when I do, I feel sick as it all feels so wrong. I feel like I have a centimetre worth of glue or papier-mâché stuck on half my head - like there is a layer of something protecting it like a shell. I shut my eyes and try and block out the dizziness and sensations while Dave washes my hair a couple of times with the shampoo. He says he has got rid of most of the glue and only a small amount of blood and scabs remain around the scar in the areas where he won't rub. I keep asking him is there glue on my scalp, to which he says "no" and I realise the numbness isn't caused from something being stuck there. It's my head causing that. I keep saying it must still be swollen and numb from the surgery. Then as he is combing with lots of conditioner and a wide toothed comb a whole wodge of glued hair falls out my head, and Dave needs to trim yet more away as he tells me it is beyond being untangled. It's horrid. The stuff of nightmares where you brush your hair and it all just starts to fall out in clumps. I get out the bath exhausted and crying as so much hair fell out and the realisation that my head doesn't have glue numbing it. The pain doesn't help, it seems that when the area is touched the pain level increases.

Crying, I manage to pull on some clothes over my hips and Dave has to dry my hair with the hairdryer as I cannot hold my hands up, nor tip my head forwards to dry my hair upside down, nor in fact dry it myself. I need to lie down again for a while after this ordeal, as I'm exhausted.

Once my hair is washed and dry and I have managed to get back downstairs and eat some lunch that Dave has made, we take some more pictures of the scar to see what it actually looks like. It oddly helps me know what I am feeling, where the scar is in relation to my numb parts of head. I still can't quite appreciate the size of it, and that the scar goes from the centre back of my neck, to well above my right ear. It's odd when you cannot see a thing as it's behind your head. Plus I can focus on a photo better, as I manage to see them ok without the small screen spinning too much, I can adjust it to where my vision feels best. I still think it's a shame it's not Halloween at the moment- I could scare a few people with a real zip in my head!

22nd May 13.51

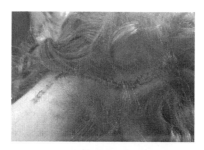
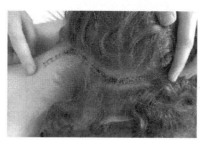

I also realise it was on the 22nd just one month ago I found out I had a tumour. Wow! That has been one long and very emotional month.

That night I slept soundly most the night for the first time in ages, only waking once for some more arnica and a glass of water. I can tell I've stopped the steroids.

Monday 23rd May. Ummm... today is the day I should have been seeing the neurologist had I just kept to the G.P referral on the NHS and not managed to get the MRI done privately. It brings it back how insane it is... I have already had a major operation done - as urgent!

In the morning (well it might have been more lunch time, as I am not getting up that early at the moment!) I decide to sit outside in the sun on my sunbed. I remind Dave to call Giggs Hill surgery up to book an appointment to get my staples removed for this Friday, as requested, with either a nurse or doctor. I hear him talking to the receptionist and querying how many staples I have. "About 40? Roughly 30 on the main scar at the back and another 7 or so on the front." Then I hear him repeating something along the lines that he will need a double appointment as they cannot manage to take that many out in one, and they don't have any double appointments left. I am livid with the surgery and so despite still struggling a little when I have to think about what I want to say and not finding it the easiest to think or talk quickly, grab the phone off of him. I ask the receptionist what he just said, and he explains that I cannot have the staples removed there as they don't have 'any' nurses or doctors free. He can book me an appointment for the following Tuesday, as Monday is a Bank Holiday.

I scream and cry down the phone at him, swearing and ranting as to just how are we supposed to book ANYTHING with their bloody useless surgery? I had BRAIN SURGERY last week, only got discharged from hospital Friday evening and today is the first day we could call the surgery, I NEED the staples removed next Friday as I have been told not to leave them in any longer. THEY are supposed to care for me and yet cannot do it. Can they do anything useful? I don't want anyone to come and visit me, I just need to see ANYONE at the surgery who can remove them. Any doctor or nurse, I have the bloody removal tool. It can't be hard to do this with 4 days' notice? When he again tells me he cannot do anything I tell him to fuck off, if I had just listened to their bloody useless doctors I would most likely be dead soon or have already had a stroke, and they cannot even do this simple thing now. I don't want to know any more. Fuck off. And slam the phone down on him. The garden continues to spin as I sit there crying as to what I can do.

Dave calls up the neurosurgery ward at St Georges and they say it is fine to go and have them removed there on Friday. Not that I need to drive there and back in one go when I am feeling nauseous before I even move, let alone being in a car for an hour's drive minimum. But at least I trust them there.

18.11. Text to Nicola

> *"Quite dizzy still and hard to focus at times- but pain going down. Just left with a large zip line on neck and head that's tightening!!"*

I am again able to reduce the painkillers a bit and only take a couple of doses a day. But the muscles in my head and neck feel like they are pulling and everything feels like it is trying to get feeling back. When I touch the back of my head, the whole of my right side feels about ½ centimetre bigger than the left hand side. The lump that was at the centre back of my head feels puffy on my right, so much so I cannot feel a lump, but on the left I can just about feel a ridge, but nothing like I did before the operation. I don't know if my head is now a different shape where the acrylic implant is, or if it is still just very swollen. In fact I don't even know how big or where the implant is. I want to know this - it is my head after all.

The days pass in a blur- they all blend into the same day of feeling dizzy and unreal, eating and sleeping. Trying to heal.

25th May 10.14 - Text to A *(howz ya zipper?)*

"Very zipped and tight! But ok, can sleep now (just waking up properly) and I can move a bit better.
Still quite dizzy at times and blurry eyes- but they said that could be a few months... and have huge numb bit that feels like something is added to my skull- but hopefully some of that is stitches pain.
But it's going in the right direction and the lump is not there... ❤ *"*

It is weird, as I really struggle to wake up now. Well I had been feeling similar for the last few months, I can wake up, talk to Dave and feel ok without even opening my eyes for 15 -20 minutes or so. I just don't realise I haven't opened them, nor feel I want or need to. When I do finally decide I need to open my eyes, it takes me several minutes to be able to focus properly. It is hard to work out focus when your world is spinning. Often I end up looking at a game on my phone or something to help me focus, otherwise I just keep dozing back off again, and again.

25th May. I see this on my Facebook newsfeed.

"A MESSAGE FOR TODAY: "The difficult situations in your life have not come to you because you deserve it. They have not come to you because you are doing something wrong. They are not a punishment. They have come to you because somewhere inside the coal, there is a diamond. That diamond is the key to the very thing you have been asking for. Your job is to sort through the coal for that diamond. And when you do find that diamond, the coal will make complete sense. You will see that the universe is not punishing you. In fact it is lining you up with the exact thing you have been wanting."

~ Teal Swan"

I hope so! I strongly feel and have always felt that this is some kind of 'positive' lesson for me. Yes when you are in it, the last thing it feels is positive, but there is a bigger picture and that is positive. That if I can get over this, I can get over anything and will have so much less fear. Maybe my joke about them taking out 'all my crap' when they removed my tumour, wasn't really such a joke. It's time to let go of all the rubbish!

It's also a week since my operation today. Only a week and yet it feels like it happened both a month ago and yesterday at the same time.

26th May 16.10

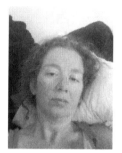

The days are taking ages, I look crap and feel crap, but keep focusing that 'this too will pass' and taking it one day (or even hour) at a time. I keep saying that I want the spinning to stop for 10 minutes. Just let me get my balance and vision back for a little while so I can recharge. So that when I am sitting I don't feel I am on a merry go round, or when I am eating it feels like I am trying to put food in my mouth while on a boat. Shutting my eyes is the only way to feel vaguely normal.

27th May. Today we drive back to St George's to get my staples removed. It's not easy being in the car for that long, even with a pillow to lean on, and several times I have to shut my eyes to stop the nausea from the spinning world causing me travel sickness even with my Sea Band's on. Although this time going there is a whole lot less scary than when Dave drove me there last. It seems we planned the journey time well, or I had my eyes shut a lot, as the traffic doesn't seem too bad. As we walk in, Dave and I have to do the now normal walking arm in arm, so I don't lose my balance. But I can now turn a little and vaguely see the cars as we are crossing, when only 2 weeks ago I couldn't turn or see them at all.

Walking back into the building, past the operating theatre and up that same damn corridor is emotional. I don't know how to describe having sadness and joy, plus fear, love and gratitude all at the same time. I guess I have been through every emotion walking into hospital, around it, into theatre and then back out of this building over the past few weeks. It is still just over a month since I first found out I even had a tumour, and 3 weeks since I first stepped foot in neurology here. We walk back down to the nurses' station and ask the first person which nurse will be able to remove the stitches. The male nurse tells me of course he can, asks why I needed to come back here and then says they are easy to remove - any nurse at my G.P. surgery could have done them. Yes, most probably, but not with the ones who I am registered with! He gets me to go and sit down on a treatment couch, while I lean my head on Dave and he pulls the staples out one by one. Occasionally I feel a sharp pinch, but I think it is when he manages to pull a bit of my hair as he is removing them. I then lean backwards and he takes the last few out of the top of my head. Done.

Part of me wants to walk into the wards and see if anyone is still there who was a patient when I was, and another part really doesn't want to see a thing. I hope a week later there will not be many people still there and so Dave and I just walk back out. We get to the car park ticket machine and it tells us we have been less than 15 minutes, so we don't have to pay for parking. Bearing in mind it probably took us a lot more than 5 minutes to walk up and down to the second floor ward, it means the staples actually being removed took less than 10 minutes. Why my local doctors' surgery could not do this, I don't know.

I get back home and want to lie down, once again I am shattered.

Posted on Facebook

> *"Staples out!*
> *Now just need it all to heal and get my balance back* ♥ *-*
> *with Dave Barlow."*

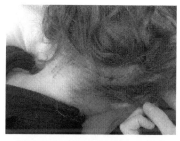

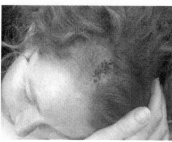

27th May. Text to A

> *"Staples out!!*

Had a good night but still feeling dizzy and walking to ward in hospital was hard, but I am getting stiller bits when I am sitting down and I can feel more normal .. ❤
slow but ok x"

Chapter 21 - I Just Did It

The next morning my neck pain seems to have ramped up the scale, I have taken paracetamol and yet every time I seem to move my neck is hurting insanely. When I walk anywhere it feels like my muscles are going into spasm, I actually have to ask Dave to walk along behind me, pushing into my neck muscles to relieve the pain a little as I can't walk anywhere without crying if he doesn't. I end up just sitting with my head to one side and crying while my Mum finds the codeine and I take one. It does seem to relieve some of the pain, but I feel nice and spaced out again, and I hate it. I really want to feel 'here', fully seated in this time and place, fully conscious and aware, not this constant feeling of being drugged, drunk, dizzy and horrid unreality.

A family friend comes to visit and despite me saying that this is worse than I felt a few days ago, she tells me that considering I had major brain surgery just 10 days ago I am looking amazing and far better than she thought. I feel awful.

I don't know if the pain increased as the staples were removed and now my body is able to move inside and start to heal better or that it takes 10 days for cut muscles to properly start to heal or what really causes it. My neck is still swollen, especially at the back right and I can feel a lump of fluid that increases and decreases at various times. I keep asking Dave if it looks any better and he tells me it seems to visibly change. The arnica cream especially soothes it, but if I lay wrong it makes it worse and more swollen again. This is one problem with leaving hospital after 2 days- there is no one to question anything or to notice if your symptoms are an issue or not.

28th May 13.02. Text to Nicola

> *"My neck muscles keep tightening right up and spasming –*
> *it's awful! Have had to take codeine purely from this pain..."*

I end up on the sofa for much of the day asleep, despite it being sunny in the garden, as it's the only way I can get comfortable and the codeine is making me feel awful. Nausea doesn't help much of anything either, I just feel in pain, grumpy and sick. The day seems to last forever.

18.26. Text to A

> *"My zip line has gone! But feeling crap and grumpy today-*
> *neck muscles really hurting and going into spasm at times* ☹
> *Ended up taking codeine too now feel super tired...*
> *I guess it's reconnecting- but shit it hurts!! X"*

29th May 11.18

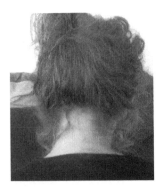

Thankfully the pain has again subsided a little, well I don't need the codeine! Although have decided I will take alternate ibuprofen and paracetamol for a few days to hopefully minimise pain and keep the swelling down. After all it has got to be better that having to re take steroids, or having a relapse as the other woman in the last ward had. As long as I take the tablets with food they don't seem to be causing me so much nausea as they did, maybe my body has got used to them or maybe I am getting used to the nausea from the constant motion sickness?

30th May. Mum again comes round and she asks me would I like to get out and watch Adam play cricket at the local club for a short while? I don't know if it's a good idea or not, if I am up to going out yet, but feel I am going stir crazy indoors and will give it a try. After all it cannot be any harder than having to leave the hospital or go back in to remove the staples, and I have done that OK. So Mum drives me to the club, round to the back of the clubhouse where I get a walking stick and walk the 20 or so metres to the pavilion.

We sit down on some chairs in the shade and attempt to watch the game. It is actually easier to look into the distance than it is to look just a few metres away as the spinning vision seems a little less obvious. In fact at times it doesn't seem much different to waking at night and your vision has not quite settled, but you still manage. However I cannot concentrate much, I cannot even sit still for long and so after half hour or so we get back into the car. It is odd, as no one asked me how I was. I don't know if I no longer look that ill now, Adam told them what I had done and they didn't want to intrude, or they were all just being too polite and didn't want to ask why I had a walking stick and looked awful!

I find it hard when people don't ask... I find it hard not to tell the world (or anyone I meet) that I am feeling pissed most of the day and night and struggling to cope with I the fact I cannot control it at all and I can do nothing else than just trust I am ok. Trust that I am healing. Trust that my tumour (the tumour that I still have not really acknowledged I had) is gone. Trust that one day I will be able to walk and see properly again, have some muscle return and energy back.

30th May 13.26. Text to A

> *"Neck stopped the spasms...slowly getting there... Vision and 'stopping spinning all the time' gradually getting better too"*

I am still not able to look at a computer screen for too long, although I am now managing to actually do the online shopping, rather than Dave reading through the items and we both decide if we need them and him having to actually order them as I can't look at the screen for more than a few seconds. But despite this, by the end of doing even a basic shopping order I am feeling decidedly travel sick still and have to lie down with a ginger tea. I can also look up more urgent information and just about manage to read it, or delete my daily emails, but I cannot use it to read a thing and help stop my boredom of TV.

I am also told that my uncle is really ill now and not responding to much. I still don't really understand it, the seeming randomness as to why someone gets ill, and lives or dies. It is far too close for comfort and confusing as to why. All I can do is send my family my love and pray that my uncle is content as he passes over into the next world.

2nd June. I think my family are now a little bored with looking after me! Dave is obviously having to work as much as he can to catch up on all the hours, phone calls and messages he has missed and so outside in his office (although we have two phones so I can page him if I need anything) and the older kids are all going about their lives. Calla still has a couple of GCSE exams to revise for and sit and Zach has his BTEC assignments to finalise. So much of the day I am here with Roan and if the weather isn't good enough to sit in the garden I am still watching that blooming TV. Somehow when it is sunny, even when I am just sunbathing in the garden the day seems to go much quicker...

19.58. Text to A

> *"Bored shitless! TV is awful, kids been out (due back any minute) Dave working...*
> *Problem is I am still dizzy and neck swollen...and it's not even been sunny....*
> *Patience...I am learning patience ❤"*

3rd June. My Uncle died this morning. I don't know what to say, although send my condolences to my family. Why, when we were both ill at similar times, is he now dead?

Later that afternoon, I read this article online: (part of it I have copied here)

> *"I just did it. I just did the Thing one day, one Saturday, and came home on Sunday after having climbed a mountain. Never doubt yourselves, please, not even once.*
> *This life thing is hard, and being here, being present... being a person, it takes courage.*

Feeling fully, loving fully... surrendering to all those possibilities, possible successes and potential failures, that takes guts, and it's scary.

Sometimes climbing a mountain is easier than making that phone call or doing the Thing.

The world is a big place, and sometimes you feel teeny tiny and small. I feel teeny tiny more often than not. But you can climb mountains, literally! You can do the Thing, whatever the Thing is.

You don't have to do it well; you don't have to do it joyfully. You don't have to shout about it and be positive and post photos on Instagram in a field of flowers smiling with an inspirational quote underneath.

You can do the Thing covered in your child's upchuck, you can do it wearing no makeup, you can do it tear-stained and smelly with a sink full of dirty dishes.

You can do the Thing scared, feeling small... teeny tiny. You can do it tired; you can do it in pain. You can do the Thing broke and depressed and lost and lonely.

Doing the Thing does not require you to be pretty, happy, excited, confident, eager, cheerful, or to have a positive mind-set.

All you actually need to have to do that dreaded Thing is a few seconds of stubbornness, enough stubbornness to try, to make a little teeny tiny small and smelly promise to yourself that you will try, that you're open to it not working and looking stupid and feeling small.

Whatever the Thing is, it is possible and you don't need to be a positive inspirational Instagramming goddess to do it. You just need good old stubborn you."

As I am reading it and for a good while after, tears stream down my face. I share the article on my Facebook page along with this:

> "Yep ... I had a major op... On a bloody brain tumour... I have felt shite after, stupidly dizzy, scared, had full panics at the hospital (mostly as I cannot stand to hear others being ill and bleeps are like alarm clocks in my head!), cried till I've run out of tears ...
> But I have done it! I fucking did it and I know that it was the love of my kids, Dave, my family and friends, as well as so many of you on here that kept me together.
> I did 'the thing' and it seems that nothing has changed ... yet everything has ♥ "

In the early evening Calla is looking at my scar line to see how it is healing, how the hair is growing back and if my head and neck looks less swollen... and notices under a patch of hair and a scab that I still have a staple left in. No! I can't have - but I do. I just feel sick and cry.

3rd June. 19.07. I ask on Facebook if anyone has any good ideas on what to do?

> "Grrrr –Calla has just seen they have left a staple in my head!
> What is the chance I can get it removed at GP surgery when

they couldn't even take them out when tried to book 5 days in advance and I now don't have the remover …

Any options but walk in clinic or A&E … And when would be a good time to go?
Either that or it's back to St George's …"

It seems the options will be go to A&E or walk in clinic and hope they have the same type of remover, or go back to St Georges. I will have to go somewhere tomorrow morning. Great.

Saturday 4th June. The rogue staple… Dave wants to just try and remove it himself! I don't know if he is joking or not, but he doesn't get the option to even look as I say it's my head and I want it removed properly.

He and I decide we don't want to sit in A&E for several hours as one extra staple left in my head won't be a priority, so decide to try the most local next option which would be the local walk in clinic. We drive to Teddington, park easily and walk slowly in the clinic. We ask the receptionist if the nurses would have any staple removers as I no longer have the correct remover (as the nurse didn't know they missed a staple and so didn't give me a remover!) She phones the nurses who tell her they do not have any staple removers at all and the only option is to go to A&E as they will have them…

So we get back in the car and have to drive almost back past our home and in the opposite direction to go to St George's. Problem is, even before we are at the roads where we would turn off to go home I am feeling stupidly travel sick. Do we continue to St George's now, or go home and try again later? I put my sea bands back on, shut my eyes and tell Dave we should just to do it now while we are in the car. I still feel nauseous when we arrive there - about an hour from when we first left the house.

This time the car park is quiet as it's a Saturday, so we park almost as we enter the car park, walk arm in arm back up to the neurology ward, feel every emotion under the sun again in the few minutes of walking through 'that' corridor and go back to the nurses station. This time we see a different nurse who asks me to follow them to the medical room while they find a remover tool. I still feel sick and want to sit down but I just tip my head forward while they pull this one staple out. We get back in the car, again in less than 15 minutes and have to drive back home. I am still sitting with my eyes mainly shut as Dave is instructed to stop while driving on a roundabout by a police motorcyclist. We then watch as a load more police motorbikes come up off the A3, so I get my phone camera out to see who it may be. Just as more police escorts arrive and a car appears with a woman wearing a blue dress inside it, so I take a picture. Dave tells me it looks like the queen, and when I enlarge the photo later, yes it appears to be the queen on her way to the Epsom Derby. If only I cared.

The next day Dave has an afternoon gig and so at 2pm leaves me here with Calla and Roan. Most of the day I am sitting outside in the garden and I feel so much better not having to look at anything too close. The sun also still feels so healing.

Somewhere in this Calla comes out telling me I need to nit comb her hair as one of her friends said they have head lice and she has an itchy head, so she thinks she does. So I end up sitting on the garden sunbed, attempting to brush thoroughly and logically the thickest, longest hair you would ever be able to fit through a nit comb, while clipping up the rest of it. It's actually almost funny, as I can barely see what I am doing, can only partly see if there are any lice, have no chance of seeing any eggs in her hair, but still continue combing. Calla tells me there are a few tiny lice and I seem to be removing them, so I just continue. About an hour later I am finished and then have to attempt cooking dinner for the first time in ages. Dave had left a roast chicken cooking, so I only have to remove it, put on the (already chopped) vegetables and make a gravy. I manage it and almost feel a little better doing things - albeit very slowly and planned.

Sun 5th June. Text to Dave

> *"Got some balance back!! Dinner is done x"*

7th June. In the evening I decide to try and get in the bath. I don't get my head wet, but I really want a soak. I feel my skin seems to need exfoliating or something as it just feels like I have an extra layer on it. It is either something actually up with my skin or that my nerves and feelings have been damaged. I also have a horrid pain, I assume from where they put the catheter in. I sit in an Epsom salt bath, rub my skin and shave my legs... and it feels so much better. I am actually able to lean my head on the back of the bath without pain. It feels odd, yes, but is not actually painful. I take a homeopathy tablet for the bladder soreness and that seems to go too.

22.06. Text to A

> *"Just managed a bath where I didn't just feel pain! Bliss!! So must be getting better ☺"*

9th June. I am finally managing to get myself up, showered and downstairs each morning, even if it could be classed as very late morning! Today Alison comes round and does a Bowen treatment on me while I sit on a chair in the garden. It is bliss as I really feel like it is helping my body relax, and feel so much straighter afterwards. (Especially as I know I have been so bent over sideways) The worst part is it is so clearly obvious how much muscle mass I have lost, on my legs I can actually see the shin bone and then the muscle falling away flat from the side of it. It reminds me of my Nan shortly before she died.

Dave calls up Mr Jones secretary about the continued swelling in my neck and what looks like fluid still there, they call back later and I am told to come back to St George's tomorrow for him to look at it.

17.21. Text to Nicola.

> "Days are very much blending into each other!! It's almost 3 weeks since I got back home but it varies between it feeling like days and weeks!
> Head and neck is still quite puffy- am back at St George's tomorrow to check- but think it can take a while to go down. Will admit it's frustrating- especially as was home so quick after op!
> Bowen really helped relax me...I know all my muscles were tight- well and gone- I can see my bones!"

Text to S.

> "My neck is still very puffy.
> I am a fair bit more mobile now- can shower by myself and everything is not such a chore- but also very much still recovering x"

Chapter 22 - Numbskull

10th June. Back to St George's today for Timothy Jones to look at the swelling in my neck. I walk into the neurology ward where they have told us to go to on the phone and Dave and I have to wait in a side room for a while. Suddenly what I thought was a routine follow up of checking my neck seems to be of a concern, but I don't know why. Then Mr Jones comes in and takes a look at my scar and head. He tells me it has healed really well and that my hair has grown really fast, but agrees that there is still a fair bit of swelling and that they will do another CT scan to see if the swelling is just on my neck from the operation (he says that when they do this operation in children it can take 6 weeks for the swelling to go) or that I will need a shunt put in place.

My mind is saying 'A what?' I have never heard of a shunt. It seems that when the fluid is wrongly draining or filling your skull they put a shunt in- which is a drainage tube from your skull straight into your gut, so the fluid can get absorbed there. I sit there thinking 'What? What the fuck? No. I am not having another operation. Please don't tell me I need one. I don't want a tube into my guts. That's not something that sounds right. Surely the fluid will mess my guts up? And stomach health is crucial to your overall health.' And just silently hoping and praying that this doesn't apply to me. Mine is just fluid that has been there since the operation. The fact I am again having another dose of radiation seems a minor concern to the thought of needing another operation.

I say I have been having a few headaches for the last couple of days, but nothing like before. I know I mention that the clicking inside my head had stopped and how I put my hand on my tailbone to relieve the noises and the pressure in my head. I say I had craniosacral therapy that really helped me before the operation, so I used what I could of that technique of moving the cerebrospinal fluid down. "That fluid is in your brain and spinal cord, right?" he nods and looks at me a little strangely. "Well I know you think this is bonkers and it might all be in my imagination that it helps, or it may have something in it, but, well, it worked for me. And I thought you might be interested to know?"

I was then asked how my head was feeling, and I mentioned that it still felt numb and like I had a layer of something on top of it, and Mr Jones explained that this would be from the cut nerve, I must have looked puzzled at him as he roughly showed me on his head where there is a main nerve and that it goes to the top of your skull, and that they had to cut it at the neck during my operation. That I would always have a numb patch although the other nerves would try and compensate in time. I feel blank. That is it, I won't be getting the feeling back when the swelling from the operation goes down as there is no nerve there. That explains it. Oh why the fuck didn't I realise this before? I want to grieve over this news, it sort of doesn't matter in the scheme of things, but I need to mourn it. Accept it. I feel a huge sob run through me, bite my lip to stop me blubbing once again and simultaneously feel a love that it really isn't important.

So he tells us we need to go to the radiology section- this time on the opposite side of the corridor to the neurology wards, and we more or less walk straight into the CT scanning room. Dave waits outside with my bag and iPod, and the radiographer asks me if I need to remove any jewellery etc. Um yes, I have 5 earrings in. Problem being they are the type you get from the body piercing salons, where you put the earring in from the back and twist a small ball at the front of your ear onto the bar. But I cannot do this twisting movement very well yet and had to get Calla to put the earrings back in for me a couple of weeks ago. I manage one reasonably well, just about manage the second and then it feels like my fingers will no longer feel let alone turn this tiny sphere. It also doesn't help when things are all a bit dizzy and you can only just see them, and certainly not clearly. Especially when I have just been told I might need another operation! I ask the radiologist can she help me remove them, struggle to explain how they are work to her and feel totally useless. It seems that when I am talking in a normal conversation, I am ok, but when I have to explain something it is really, really hard to do. I get my words muddled up and say things the wrong way round (sometimes I don't even realise). She finally twists off the earring fronts, then she drops one of the balls on the floor. She can't see it, I have no hope of seeing it, so I say not to worry we will get another. The rest of them are loose in a small tray she has given me. (I cannot put the front back on the stem easily, even when they are not on me)

Thankfully I don't need to do anything else as I have no other metal on my clothing and so get in the scanner. I say my silent prayer to the angels to make it OK, that I won't need a shunt and that the operation scars all look like they are healing well. I am definitely grateful CT scans are only a few minutes long as they are not the most comfy things, even with the neck and head supports. I get back outside to Dave with my tray of jewellery and spend a few minutes trying to reconnect them so I can put the whole earrings in my purse and hopefully not lose any more.

We go back and sit in the room we came from to wait...

I can't even think about needing a shunt, about another operation, so I don't. I can't think about my cut nerve. I simply play a game on my mobile phone and almost sit in silence as I don't want to even talk to Dave. I don't want to express me to myself, let alone him, and certainly not a Doctor. After half an hour or so another doctor arrives to tell us the scan was fine, there is no extra fluid around the brain, it's just the fluid from the operation and the headaches are as all the membrane etc has been moved during op and is thinner and more sensitive than normal. I am told more water and rest...we can go home. Phew! Although somehow I felt I knew that.

As we walk back downstairs Dave tells me he needs the toilet, so I wait leaning on a wall right by the main neurology entrance as Dave walks off down the corridor following the toilet signs. Then I see Mr Jones walking towards me from the same corridor Dave walked down. He comes over and confirms with me that my scan was great, that there is no extra fluid, the swelling looks good and the area where the tumour was is healing nicely. He explains again that I will continue to be dizzy for a while as the area the tumour was had pushed into my brain and it will take a while for things to move back into this space. I laugh and say – "Well and I probably have a little brain missing- but I accept you only took my negative parts!" And "Yes I am really dizzy, but it seems to be getting a little better the last few days". At this point Dave comes back out, and he quickly explains that he is pleased to him. It's odd talking to someone who has just saved your life. So I just smile and say goodbye.

As I get back in the car, Dave tells me Mr Jones secretary had mentioned that they may have had to put a shunt in when she spoke to him on the phone, and that he realised when they got there that the doctors had already set it up to do so if I needed it. I am slightly annoyed that he didn't even warn me, but... it's not much point getting stressed over it now. I don't need it and that's all that matters.

11th June. On Facebook -

> *"Can any of my lovely friends send me any more healing, good vibes, prayers or anything positive please?* ❤ ❤
>
> *I have had headaches again as well as swelling on my neck and head which hasn't gone down since op... I had ct scan yesterday and it's all ok (thankfully no swelling on brain or I would have needed another op for a shunt !) but I could really do with starting to feel more normal again.*

The dizziness is also slowly improving daily ... Which is bliss
♥

*And everyone I am sure helped get me out of hospital so
quick ... So thank you xxx"*

12th June. This might explain why I had been having headaches
again. I have light bleeding starting (I assume start of period) even if
it's just over 3 weeks after a brain tumour operation. Once again (as
before the op) I have a stupidly bad headache. I am back on
paracetamol and ibuprofen too - and it doesn't fully touch it...
assume I just have to lie down and accept? It just feels like another
thing I cannot cope with.

Chapter 23 - Beautiful Scars

14th June. Zach is playing a few songs with his college band outside the college today, I really want to go to and see him and support him, and try to get a bit ready to go. But I can't manage it, my headache is still too painful – it feels like my sinuses may explode and it hurts every time I lean, or bend down. Plus I am too dizzy to stand around for long and I don't think I could walk as far as I would have to getting from the car park into the college. I don't want it to be obvious and make a scene if I feel worse or need to leave. I guess I am scared of doing too much. I sit at home and cry a bit more.

15th June. Posted on Facebook.

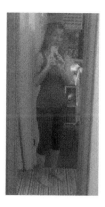

"Hey almost back to where I was ... ❤
Still a bit headachey and still have a swollen neck and can't turn that well ...
But I can have a shower, my vision and balance is returning and I have long hair again and even the shaved lines aren't as obvious !

Hopefully a few more weeks and it will be like before this started ... ♥ ♥ ♥
Albeit with a fuck off great scar, a numb patch and a couple of shave lines! .. ☺
♥ ♥ ♥ ♥ ♥ ♥ ♥ ♥ ♥ ♥ "

I find it quite funny really... on the outside no one seems to know a thing, certainly not that I had brain surgery less than a month ago. They don't even seem to notice that I am dizzy, I guess I have mostly stopped the falling or walking into things since the operation. Yet, on the inside, everything has changed... Everything.

17th June. Today is my Uncle's funeral. The crematorium is booked for 9.30am and it is at least a 75 minute drive away on a normal day without the rush hour traffic. I know I cannot be awake and ready in time to leave here at 8am and then still function for the rest of the day, as much as I would like to be able to. So I have let my Auntie know that I will be getting to the venue after the service as I do want to see my family there. I must be getting a little better with coordination and vision as I manage to put on a bit of mascara for the first time in ages, and actually see what I am doing. We leave just after 9am and I don't actually feel too nauseous on the drive- although it is still somewhat uncomfortable to sit and lean my head. As we arrive at the pub, so do all the cars that have just left the crematorium. I feel a bit awkward as I see several of my family who I have not seen since I was ill, let alone after the operation, and so they ask me how I am. They seem pleased I am looking so well when the operation was a month ago tomorrow. When they see the photos of the scar and staples they seem even more so. But at a funeral seems the wrong time to be too positive and happy I have survived. Or maybe it is the exact time you need to feel positive and happy for those still alive? I don't know. However both my auntie and cousins say that my uncle would have wanted me to be well again after, and are so pleased that I am. It just feels a little too close for comfort.

While I am there I realise I am so much less dizzy now, although I have to sit down most of the time I can manage to walk into the toilets alone and not feel I will fall over, even walk up a down a couple of steps without support as long as I concentrate when I need to step and do it carefully. I cannot stay too long and we leave about 2pm. I am shattered and feel my eyes are twitching from exertion. It is the most I have done in ages. I go home and fall asleep on the sofa.

20th June. Today I manage to go to Kingston College for their album release with two of Zach's songs in it. It is not exactly that exciting as its more of a College event than for him, but I so want to be able to do something to celebrate his last year there and of getting both good grades and amazing songs written over the last couple of years. I still have to hold Dave's arm when we walk too far, but I feel I am finally getting there and the dizziness is manageable now. I don't know what people think, or if they even notice? But it is still hard to deal with.

21st June. 20.11. Calla takes a picture of my scar, with her finger on the top part of it, and tells me it is both really fading and my hair is covering the rest really well.

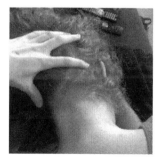

I realise this quote that I found at the Creative Day back in April is very much true, and has now taken on a different meaning. Yes. I survived!

> *"We must see all scars as beauty. Okay? This will be our secret. Because take it from me, a scar does not form on the dying. A scar means, "I survived."*
> — *From Little Bee: A novel, Chris Cleave*

22nd June. Today I have some more Bowen. It feels it is really helping, and finally I am able to lay down flat on the couch and Alison can treat near my scars. I feel so much more balanced after.

Calla again takes some photos of my neck for me, it's so odd to have a scar you can never actually see.

Posted on Facebook.

> *"The scar - tho been told it looks darker on the photo*
> *Getting used to the numb bit of my head and gradually able to do normal stuff again. Albeit slowly and more tired easily*
> *X*
> *But 6 months of dizziness has all but gone!!!* ♥♥♥ ☺ *"*

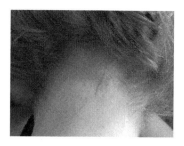

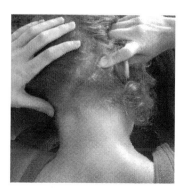

I have been dizzy for six whole months. Half a year! I don't think unless you have ever experienced this just how much it means to be able to feel ok again. To sit and look at anything without it moving or spinning, thinking that you will fall off your seat when you are firmly sitting on it, bumping into walls, tables, chairs, doors and people almost every single time you walk, having to walk with your arms wide to keep your balance when you do, eating when it feels like you are on a merry go round and can't find your mouth. The only respite when you have your eyes shut and are laying down. No wonder I am shattered. Every cell of me is exhausted. Yet the nightmare is finally going. Unless I am tired I no longer feel dizzy, wobbly, off balance or spinning. I can shut my eyes standing up and stay there! I never thought I would be able to cope with this, but I have. I did it. I survived what I didn't think I could.

25th June. Dave and Zach are playing a gig in Kingston. Mum says she will take me there, so I don't have to go early when Dave leaves. I am still a little worried if I will be able to listen to the music when it is loud, as I had really not been able to do so before I had surgery, but Mum says she will pick me up again at any time and the pub is quite large so know there are places where it is much quieter to sit. I arrive there before they start to play and sit down on the sofa at the end of the room while they are setting up. Some couple with a youngish child were about to leave but as they are getting sorted start to talk to me about the band. I tell them it's my husband and son playing, they then mention that I don't look old enough to have an 18 year old son and ask how old I am. I say I am 42 and they both tell me I don't look it. To which I start laughing and tell them I take that as a total compliment as only a few weeks ago I had brain surgery and it's been the hardest time of my life. If I no longer look ill that is a good start and for them to say I don't look my age is amazing. They both seem quite shocked and say they never would have guessed. It feels so odd - I still don't quite get it myself! And I honestly don't know if they are lying or not.

When the band start playing I sit right at the back of the pub, almost around the corner of a wall so that they are obscured and realise that I am ok with the noise, so gradually as different friends enter I move forwards and even end up at one point standing just a couple of metres away from the PA speakers. It is so good to finally be able to go back out and be 'normal' again. Listen to the music I am used to and love, have a laugh with others. At a few points I really notice the numbness in my head, it seems worse when I touch my hair, or it catches in my handbag on my shoulder. Then I just feel I have a wig attached to half my head and the numbness is noticeable even when I am not touching any part of it. But I don't feel dizzy, a few unreality feelings at times, but nothing that I can't cope with. I stay there until the end, and even manage to carry a guitar case back to the car when I leave to go home.

29th June. I decide to get a haircut. I did trim about 3 inches off the back myself before I knew I was having the operation, but my hair is a mess and I have short bits in it at both the front and back. I get to the hairdressers and they manage to wash my hair over the sink with an extra neck support. The hairdresser has known me for the last 20+ years and so he knows how infrequently I have my hair cut, and also why I am having it cut so there are no awkward conversations about it. The consensus with the three hairdressers is to leave the short patches as you won't see them that well in my long curly hair, so I agree to just have a few inches cut off it, hope it helps with the numbness feelings, and for it to remove any dried knotty hair. It is the oddest feeling when someone is fiddling with my hair… it seems to accentuate the total numbness and by the end most of my head feels numb and the layer of 'papier-mâché' is even bigger than normal. I guess I need to keep touching it more often to try and improve the nerve receptors in my scalp? At that point onwards I start combing my hair much more when I am in the shower with the wide toothed comb - to try and change the sensations I am feeling.

2nd July. Written to a friend.

> "I have been feeling really tearful on/off since op, and feel I should know what to do, but can't seem to work it out! Not helped that I need more time to think than normal…but I am MUCH better than I was, and the dizziness has finally gone - after 6 months ☺ x
>
> I have at times taken staphysagria (a homeopathic remedy) as I know I have felt violated from op … but I am not sure if this is even the right remedy? …I keep saying "it's wrong" (my head, the whole op- not the remedy!)
>
> My head still feels odd…totally numb in places and like I have a load of hard glue over some of my skull and a wig on

in places. Plus at times my neck gets really tight both at the back, where they cut, and what feels like near my windpipe ☹

Dave just keeps saying "you are alive, it doesn't matter"... and while I fully get what he is saying I am still mourning what I have lost and understanding what happened... I need to offload it somehow- I still don't really get that I had a large tumour (even though I saw it clearly on MRI) much less how I caused it- or was it just really 'one of those things' and was nothing I did?? (I have seen somewhere that hemangioblastoma's are caused when the blood vessels 'develop' wrong- so could something have been there since conception??)

But I am now getting there... I can see straight, move my neck again- without pain, and don't feel drunk 24/7 ... although I am still a bit clumsy and get tired far easier than before.

I also seem to have lost my panic mode... it is far less than last year ♥ *Fight or flight reflex is said to be in the cerebellum and I wondered before op if that was what was making me so anxious!! Xx"*

9th July. Dave and Zach are playing a support slot at an outside gig in Essex. It's about a 2 hour drive away and although they start playing at 7.30pm, they need to be there for 3.30 for sound check. We collect two of Zach's friends and so have a car full. Dave has to drive through busy traffic just to get on the M25, but we manage to still arrive on time. People kept asking me how I was now, to which I don't really know how to reply but say 'I'm getting there' and thank them for asking. I still feel a little odd and tired, things can often just feel too much, plus am often struggling with finding the words I want to say which seems worse when its people I don't know that well. I don't know how much of it they notice, but I feel like I am more than a little slow and muddled at times. But hey, I have an excuse!

I am sitting with Zach's friends while they sound check – and feel it is pretty loud. I am still a little worried that something like this may trigger me to have a fit. I know I have been told I will always be more prone to them than most people, but try to put that worry to the back of my mind- and yet also avoid getting too near the speakers. Just before they start to play, the park fills up with well over 1000 people, and so our two picnic rugs are now surrounded by others with drinks in bottles and glasses, food, chairs, mats – not to mention young kids- everywhere. I wish I had put the rugs near the edge of the park now, so I don't have to walk through people. However, when I go and take pictures of the band and walk back to the rug, I actually feel I can manage it. Yes I still have to imagine in advance where I am going and check that the path is wide enough, but I don't walk into anyone, stand on or knock over anything I shouldn't and my handbag doesn't whack a small child in the face or anything awful without me even realising! I might feel a little wobbly inside, but I am so immensely grateful that I am not walking like a drunk still. If only I didn't sound like one when I spoke sometimes... especially when I am tired, and it is far too easy for me to get tired.

Chapter 24 - Back to Reality

14th July. We decide we are going to go to Dave's dad's caravan in Norfolk for a break. We went there last year a few times and enjoyed it, but I am a bit nervous about being a 3 hour drive away from home, forgetting something I need, being unable to drive, having to deal with my tiredness, sore head, sore neck and just that I struggle with organising, with thinking.

Although at the same time a huge part of me just wants to get away from surburbia and just go somewhere quiet. In fact I have been craving quiet since having my operation done... it literally feels my head is screaming to me that I need to get away from here and move somewhere with fields and trees, where I can have my own vegetable garden to grow my own food and not just containers... somewhere where I cannot hear cars on the road even at night and don't have a lorry or car pulled up outside my garden wall with the engine on several times a day, where I can see the stars at night as the sky is dark and not lit by a million street lights...

... and well, the caravan in a nice remote part of Norfolk, surrounded by nature and beaches and is far better than home is for this.

16th July. But being here is tough too, I can manage one trip a day, but that's it. If we walk on the promenade and then down the beach to the sea front and back I am exhausted. Like fall asleep in the back of the car exhausted. Physically worn out. Also my head seems to feel number after- a mix of the wind in my hair and tiredness. Plus if I still lean on it wrong, it feels like I have a plate digging in my head from the back to the side of my right ear that doesn't go off for half an hour or so at best. When I wake in the morning my neck, into my head, also seems far more sore and numb than at home, I have to lay for a while as I wake and help it release. Not that I can open my eyes for 10 or 15 minutes after waking yet anyway!

Just walking around (distances that were fine last year), even to the club house are suddenly so tiring, and I need to keep staying at the caravan and sleeping. But it's quiet and relaxing... and sunny!... and I so need this to heal me.

17th July. It is our 19th wedding anniversary while we are here. 19 years. The first family birthday or anniversary since I had this operation. I wouldn't be here without it now. It's too tough to even think about, what it would be like for the others today if I didn't have the option of brain surgery...

But as quiet as it is, after a few days of doing far more than I did when I was at home, I can feel I am getting more and more tired, probably as I am not able to nap in the day. I cannot sleep late as the lightness and birds start to wake me at 5am, so by 8.30 it feels like you have had a lie in and I do feel more refreshed than at home. (I can happily sleep until 10.30 or so at home) and Dave's dad comes to join us for our last few days here. But although he is not a pain, I can't deal with it, I can't deal with anything easily nor more than I am used to.

19th July. Posted on Facebook.

> "In the caravan on a week away... No wifi ☺ and no mobile bandwidth either ... So hence no emails or reading this much!
> But I keep waking up early - 2 hours earlier than at home- and still feeling refreshed... wonder how much it's related to being wi-fried in surburbiton?
> Think I'm moving to the countryside ...."

Then when they are all fishing (I don't fish, I just sit on the bank at the side of the lake, relax, read and sometimes watch them) someone catches a fish and tries to unhook it near to where I am sitting. As the hook was blowing in the wind I grab it (I don't want a hook blowing into my face or head) and say loudly to not pull the fishing rod as I have the hook in my hand... but Dave's Dad does and with a sharp pain I realise the hook is halfway into my thumb. The pain hurts but goes once I unhook myself, yet the main issue is I am so pissed off. Why are they holding a fishing rod with a hook on it dangling near my head... my head, I can't feel it properly, so wouldn't even know if I was hurting it and its had more than enough trauma this year... Why did he grab the line when I said I was holding it...actually why I am even here with them fishing? I hate it- just sticking hooks in a fish's mouth for fun. So I swear at him to stop being a fucking idiot, buckets of tears in my eyes, stomp back off to the car contemplating driving back to the caravan... I know I don't have a driving licence, but apart from crossing one road I will be on private property, but it's a caravan park, and I don't know if I can drive ok, how my coordination is... and I don't want to risk hurting anyone. So I just sit and sob my heart out in the back of the car while cuddling the dog.

Posted on Facebook.

> "My patience has gone... Maybe as I wanted, and thought, I was getting a relaxing break away...
> An 'after the shit' time away...
> Lost it big time ...
>
> "Problem is it seems others just continue to cast me as 'a stroppy redhead' rather than someone who just wants peace and quiet and to be able to recover from having her head opened ... ☹
> I don't want the piss taken out of me, I am healing in the sun (and I'm not even pink so I can't be fucking burning...) and I

don't find a caravan park club house entertaining! ☺
The house away from all with its own organic garden is
calling more than ever.... ❤

And I cannot stop crying...."

Whilst I don't know many things, I do know some things that help or heal me (sun, peace, kindness) and things that are just too much - bordering on torture (awful music, too much noise, violence, TV programmes) and I know I now have to address them. Let others know when it's not right for me.

Just please... why can't people listen to me? Why won't I really tell others what I think rather than bottle it all inside? Why do I just not listen to myself so much of the time? If I had I would have stayed inside and just rested today. As I am scared of being alone still that's why... Like I haven't quite been able to say the brain tumour feels like the result of 'others doing my head in' ... not listening to me. Not that we can do much if we did listen to my inner callings. We don't have money to move, or travel...or do anything much really.

But I know I have to find the balance with listening to my intuition and not hurting others feelings. Say it tactfully. Maybe today I blew... I needed the quiet too much to cope with anything else... but I do need them to listen and I need a better way. I need to be true to me.

"Coming home later... Had enough ... The garden is more
relaxing ..."

So on the 20th we leave to come back home- early. We arrive back to the mess three teenagers and one twenty something year old have made when they weren't yet bothering to tidy as they didn't expect us back for another two days... at 11.30pm I am standing by the sink washing up others mess – tears just running down my face.

Being away from home I have broken the habit of the last few months of not being able to walk the dog at all. I realise that if he doesn't pull I can walk him without it hurting me too much, my balance is finally good enough and I have the strength, so I think I am ok to manage a lap of the local park. So once we are back home I decide I am walking Enzo again at what was his normal walk time. I manage to cut the corners of the park, but walk most of the lap and I am not too shattered afterwards, and the peace of going out to the park alone is very much needed. After a couple of days I meet up with some of the regular dog walkers who are frequently there - they had assumed I had suddenly moved as they hadn't seen me since April, nor Enzo with Dave or the kids. Normally they walked him in the afternoon or evenings - very different times to what I had done. So we have some shocked conversations about me being right that I had something wrong, how bad Giggs Hill surgery was, (some of them had moved from there too!) how good St. George's was etc. But none of them knew until I told them, apparently I look 'normal'!

And yet again, doing something simple seems the hugest achievement. I almost want to walk up to people that I don't see very often while walking their dogs, or even strangers, and tell them I had major brain surgery just two months ago. That I am sorry I can't walk fast right now, sorry if my dog is super excited to be going back out for a regular morning walk and so sniffing their dog, and everything else in the vicinity, like mad. That, despite this, I am happy to be able to walk him round here, by MYSELF, something that many a time I wondered if I would ever be able to do again.

23rd July. Today I go with Dave to one of his gigs, I haven't seen the other band members in one of his bands since I was ill. It is good to get out again and the pub is set out in such a way that I can sit at the side of where Dave is playing, so he can see that I am ok and yet I don't get deafened from the speakers, so it feels ok going there even if no one else I know that well turns up and I end up sitting alone. However I feel a little odd going back to this venue as this was the pub where I first really knew there was something wrong when I felt so 'drunk' walking up the stairs. Then a friend we haven't seen for several years' turns up, so I am able to have a good catch up chat and sit with him and his sister- and still sit at the side of the band so Dave can see me. He also had not seen Dave play before, so it always seems to surprise people that he really can play guitar well! But once again it seems so very, very, odd to be talking about me looking really well, and that others wouldn't know I had brain surgery, and certainly not just two months ago. People can't see my scars, they are hidden in my hair and so they don't seem to notice. Plus, even if I still don't have the best balance, or start saying the wrong words, people just assume I am in the pub after all and have had a few drinks! ... but despite them thinking I look fine, I still need to process all that has happened, and I am most certainly not there yet.

26th July. Last week my cousin's young son had an operation at Great Ormond Street Hospital and he and his parents are all having to stay there for three weeks after the operation for his physiotherapy, and I want to go and see both my cousin and her son. I know it's no fun being in hospital, let alone for 3 weeks. I don't really fancy going there by myself yet and am not sure how much I can manage the walking and not being able to rest if I need to, and I am a little scared I could still trigger an epileptic fit if I am too worn out or something, so I take Adam with me. Somehow I manage to get there alright and be able to stand at the side of his bed for most of the couple of hours we are there. Adam entertains him by them firing nerf guns at each other and the curtains around the bed, and my cousin says how much he loves it as he enjoys having a younger person to mess around with. Once again a couple of the nurses look in amazement when they find out I had a brain tumour removed in May. As he also had neurological surgery, my cousin says she was chatting to one of the neurosurgeons about my surgery and he again was totally surprised that I was allowed home after two days, as it is just not heard of. It's still odd, as I just cry each time someone mentions surgery, I cry at how my cousin and son are, how grateful they are for the surgery. The things it has improved for him already. How much I never thought I would have had this done to me.

29/7/16. I know I am feeling grumpy, but I am struggling with this badly some days- just accepting the surgery, accepting the side effects. I didn't want them, I don't feel I deserved them. I have always tried to look after myself...so why did I get this? It seems like I cannot think about much else during the day at the moment as the feelings I am getting in my head are constantly reminding me.

I send a message to a friend.

> "I can't remember if I am repeating myself ... but the whole of today (and it seems every other day or so for a while at least) my head just feels numb....like I have laid on it and made a part numb. From the scar to the top, extending to my ear. My hair feels like a wig, and as much as I stretch my neck etc it doesn't seem to go off. The only thing that can help is laying down on my left side for a while. Dave says it's better than being dead... but its shite, and I cannot

concentrate on anything else. I feel grumpy and fed up. I didn't ask for this. I eat well and try and avoid pollutants etc to stop this type of stuff, and want to cry (and am, while writing this) I can deal with it when it only feels numb to touch...but when you can feel it all the time it is just hard. Sorry to be a pain, but it might describe it better? xx"

Chapter 25 - Getting My Head Around It

28th July. Today is a day I am not looking forwards to. I have a load of appointments at St George's to test if I have the possibility of the genetic syndrome - von Hippel–Lindau. (or VHL) I have to have my eyes checked, a kidney scan, then see a geneticist and have bloods taken. That doesn't bother me, the actual tests don't bother me, nor really does the thought that I may have something somewhere else that needs operating on in the future as I have already been told the worst of it is the tumour in the cerebellum (although I don't want another operation) … but what is really scaring me and puts my own concerns into nothing is that it is genetic and the thought I could pass this to my kids…

As it is we get there perfectly on time – just 5 minutes before the appointment as we had a rather long walk around the outside of the building. Possibly not helped that I cannot eat at all today until after the kidney scans… and that is not until after 3pm. Yet the eye clinic is running slow, I finally see someone for the basic tests after a couple of hours, only about 40 minutes before my next appointment at another clinic, so they agree that they won't have time to see me for the full eye tests before this appointment is due. Although they tell me that until the blood tests were introduced the eyes were the main diagnosis for VHL. She tells me that if I had anything showing they would laser the blood vessels. To which I breathe a sigh of relief and say 'that's ok then' and she laughs - as apparently all the patients who have had a brain tumour removed say that about laser eye surgery!

We leave there and go off to the genetics appointment, agreeing we will be back when we can. The geneticist is helpful and explains a little about why and what they are testing and what VHL does. She also explains that if I have it, that it could have started with me and there doesn't have to be a family history of similar (which thankfully there isn't) but then each of my children would have a

50% chance of having VHL as Dave doesn't need to be a carrier too. 50%. Fuck. That's too high. That means the odds are that two of my four children would have it. My mind is racing 'Would it be the ones who look more like me? What would I say to them? What would I say to whoever had it? What would I say to those that didn't? What would they say to each other? Would they hate me? Would it ruin their lives? How can my kids who play guitar amazingly expect to continue when a tumour in their cerebellum effects their coordination? The same with Adam who coaches cricket... he needs coordination and balance for that. I can't cope with even the thoughts that I may ruin what they all love most. I just can't stop them doing what they are amazing at and love'. Yes, I do sort of know I would not be actively ruining it for them, but it sure feels like it. 'I' would have given it to them. I feel a little bit sick and just start to pray that they don't see anything today.

We then have to go off to have the bloods taken as apparently they stop doing them at 3pm. (about 10 minutes) Dave leaves me there while he speaks to the scan department to say I will be a bit late and they say they will be there until 4.30. Thankfully there is hardly anyone else there as it's the end of the clinic and so I get the blood done really quickly.

We go back to the eye clinic and the Ophthalmologist scans my eyes and tells me that they look totally normal nor are there any signs for VHL, but they will still test me every 2 years for a while to check.

As the scan department also close not long after we quickly go up back there next to get my kidney scan. Again as it's near the end of the clinic we go straight in and the woman ultrasounds my belly for a while and tells us that she cannot see anything on my kidneys, but she can see what looks like a birth mark, a haemangioma, on my liver. She tells us that she doesn't think it is related to VHL, but that she will let Mr Jones and the geneticist know as it may be connected. Great. What is wrong with my liver? Is that why I have always said I don't process toxins very well?

As we finally leave the hospital, despite feeling a little nauseous, I am eating the sandwich I made hours earlier as we walk back to the car park…I am starving. I'm also thinking positive, I won't have VHL, my kids don't deserve that.

30th July. I really cannot get my head around having a brain tumour, nor getting out of hospital so quickly, nor not having any 'obvious to others' injury remaining. It also seems this is close to what other people think. As today I went to an outside festival, with a few bands playing organised by one of the pubs Dave plays at, and from the 15 - 20 people I knew there they all seem to be amazed that I look quite normal. Most of them had seen my scars on my or Dave's Facebook profiles, so knew how large the operation scar was, yet they said they cannot even see it. I had several comments that I am amazing. Amazing? I didn't really do anything, I just kept going. What other option did I have?

A friend took this picture for me as she said she really couldn't see a thing.

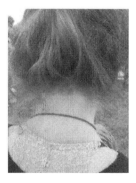

4th August. I go back for some craniosacral therapy for the first time since surgery, and it is brilliant. My head feels so relaxed – for the first time in months. At the end Paul tells me that at the start of the session it felt like my head had been hit with a frying pan, but now it feels much better and I am responding really fast to treatment. I can feel the difference, even though just after he stops my head feels horrendously tight and like the muscles are all pulling, a short while after this when I am back home my head all seems to feel much more 'normal' again. So much so I book another appointment for next week.

8th August. I am still wanting to find out the possible reasons for getting a brain tumour. As I believe like many alternative therapists that there is either a physical or emotional cause for 'most illnesses'. Although it may be just if you really listen to the reason and experience you will be taught a lesson that you needed to learn. I can't really relate to the statement 'it is one of those things', that doesn't make sense to me, unless the reason was for me to learn a lesson from it?

I was introduced this year to a concept called 'German New Medicine' and I will be honest, I have not read up too much on it, but it works with the fact that most illnesses have a 'conflict' and that it is often not in the area of the current problem. So I ask them on a group:

> *"What is the GNM reason for a hemangioblastoma? And what is cerebellum linked to?"*

The reply from an experienced practitioner is *"Dr. Hamer doesn't have anything specific about cerebellar hemangiomas. However, anything to do with the blood vessels is a self-devaluation. Since the brain itself does not experience this kind of conflict with respect to "itself", after all it is the control centre, it is entirely possible that a "local" self-devaluation occurred. In other words a physical injury to the cerebellum."*

An injury? This is the first person to say this, and I slipped and fell while standing in the bath and hit my head in almost exactly the same place a few years back! (I didn't mention this to them- just asked the questions above) I am so confused as to if this is a possibility. The surgeon didn't think this was a reason, but then he is a mainstream medical person, he probably wouldn't believe in this. And I can bet they don't ask people who have these tumours 'did they hit it?' Yet it felt connected enough for me to ask him before the operation. At the time I fell I clearly remember sitting in the bath, grateful I didn't knock myself unconscious, and yet having a funny feeling that I would somehow remember this. Plus I hit in in the exact same spot. And I would so much rather this as a possible reason for having a Hemangioblastoma and not the fact I might have von Hippel–Lindau syndrome. Although I don't really know how accurate GNM is, whilst I really believe a traumatic event can cause symptoms in a person, they seem to have a lot of possible reasons and that just acknowledging the trauma doesn't fully heal it. It is somewhat confusing.

10th August. We finally get the referral appointment with the Neuro-physiotherapists at St George's hospital. I am given the basic stretch exercises the physiotherapists told me to do after the operation and also I am made to look at a large spot on a sheet (or something else that's fixed) in front of me whilst turning my head from side to side and then when moving my head up and down. I feel useless, I can't seem to move my head smoothly and it feels after a few turns I am going the wrong way or not turning it properly. I also feel a bit dizzy again, which makes me feel tearful. Why me? Everyone else in here is about 20- 40 years older than I am. It doesn't make sense. I am also supposed to stand on a cushion and close my eyes, making sure I am next to something to keep my balance if I need to hold on. Again it is just stupid how bad I am, I feel so useless at it. Although I know I already have much more balance than just a few weeks ago... I need to retrain my brain.

Posted to friend. (After receiving letter in post from hospital today)

"Want to talk to someone who will listen...
I had tests recently to check for von Hippel–Lindau disease as
I was told I had about a 30% chance of having it due to the
brain tumour.
Anyway I needed a kidney scan and obviously they must
have scanned liver too as she said 'I have what looks like a
birthmark on my liver... And mentioned she didn't think it
was connected ...
But in my letter (I have just received) it says hemangioma ...
Which from what I can see online is related. And in which
case I have 2 markers for VHL and so I have the genetic
screw up...
And then the kids have a 50% chance each of also having
it....

I HOPE I have got it wrong and that it isn't connected ... I am
so confused with it.

Not to mention that I still have a numb head and what feels
like a wig and glue on parts of my head. Yes I know I'm alive
and I might not have been ... But I still haven't really taken it
in that I had this brain tumour!
Dave doesn't understand why I keep mentioning it, the
numbness or in growing hair pain etc. He thinks it's gone and
I am ok so it's all over. Maybe it is, but it's not gone in my
head... It's still very raw. And now this possible disease???
(How do you turn off the gene for something if it's already
happening???)
So can I just cry on you.....? X"

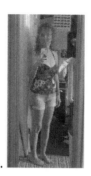

"It's almost 3 months since my op, and since I posted a picture taken in the same place of me feeling shite. (The day before I went into hospital)

But it's odd, as I probably now look the same to you as I did a year ago… I'm back to my old weight, my hair doesn't show the scars, I have stopped falling over and can turn my neck again! … But it's still like everything has changed. Some for bad (I would love to be able to feel my head again properly and it not feel tight, tender …or just wrong) but some is good. I know I don't sweat the small stuff as much anymore, I appreciate every hug (well and everything and everyone!) and just the fact my body works now and I don't feel drunk!!! And I still cry and the drop of a hat… (that can be both good and bad! ☺)

And the other thing that is odd … Is that I don't do hospitals, Dr's or even conventional medicine (I had more pharma in a week than the 20 years previously!) but yet I know I had no choice but to have this major operation. Totally scary, but no choice.

Thank you all for holding me up when I couldn't do it myself. And thank you all for your comments, support and love that healed ♥ and those that did that bit extra- thanks xXx ♥ "

Chapter 26 - Technically Normal

18th August. Today I am back for my three month follow up appointment with Timothy Jones. I sit in the waiting room looking around at a room full of people very much older than me - many of them looking far more ill. Once again I feel this is so wrong, that I don't fit in here. Not that I want to fit into a neurology department.

This time I am not having a panic attack, and when my name is called I can even walk to the consultation room without support. As I walk in Mr Jones says "You look a lot more normal", and then almost instantly laughs, "Or maybe you can't be classed as normal, but normal for you!" I laugh back and say "Yes, 'normal' would be an insult."

But he looks at my scar, tells me it has healed really well and he is pleased with it. Checks the deep hole at the front of my head as I ask is the depth of it ok and says yes, I still have a bit of room left before I could touch my brain! He says all looks good so far with the genetic tests and that he isn't concerned over the hemangioma on my liver and tells me that a hemangioma on your liver is very common, that about 10% of all people would have similar but wouldn't know as it doesn't cause any issues. He again says he thinks the hemangioblastoma would be unlikely to be genetic as I am of the right age to get one that isn't (genetic would most likely be younger), but he was still waiting on the confirmation from the blood tests and tells me I will be having a follow up MRI in November, and it will probably be with his department; although 'if' it was genetic the genetics team do all the follow up.

He again explains that I will be able to drive after 6 months, that I should be fine now as I have not had an epileptic fit and most happen shortly after the operation, but that I will always be more prone than others to having a seizure as in the right circumstances anyone could have a fit and my tolerance would always be lower than an average person.

I ask him if he really just let me go home as I was moaning about being there too much and being too awkward, and he says "No, I can't do that, you had just reached all our targets. I expected you in for a week, leaving after 2 days just doesn't happen."

He then tells me "This may seem very odd to say about having major surgery, but that you really should be proud of your achievement, you did so well' … and the floodgates open in my eyes again. I laugh again that one day I will see him without crying!

As I leave, I tell him "I know you think I am a little mad, but I did get out of here in 48 hours and I think that counts for something, so just in case anyone else ever uses homeopathy after surgery (including lots of Arnica) and also has a fast healing… please look at it again. Oh and please get in some ginger tea for nausea after the operation and manuka honey for the throat pain (from the tube down your throat) for other patients." He smiles and says that yes there are several studies to say how much ginger helps and he will see if he can get any in. I don't know if he, or the NHS, would even consider it or thinks there may be something in what I am saying… but I have to tell him. I need to start being honest and true to me.

As I leave the door and we shake hands I want to give him a hug. I am toying up in this instant if hugging your brain surgeon is an acceptable thing and decide it's probably not and just a little too honest! I leave with another 'thanks' and a crooked smile.

I actually walk out of the hospital smiling again.

Posted on Facebook.

> *"Yeah!!! ☺ I am technically normal again! ☺ (although surgeon and I agreed it's only normal for me- real normal would be an insult! ☺) just had my 3mth follow up and surgeon is really pleased, and yes he let me out 48hrs after op as I had recovered so well (he said he expected me in for a week)*
> *as he said I should be proud and more chilled and also have a sense of 'achievement'! ...he knows me more than he thinks ☺ "*

23rd August. Written to friend.

> *"Thought I would update you … surgeon didn't seem to think the haemangioma on my liver was related to the brain tumour and the possibility of VHL☺*
>
> *I still have not got the blood tests back yet (and he seemed to say they were more conclusive than we understood from other Doctor) but that basically even if it was positive I had already had the worst of what could happen! And if then the kids had it too, they would pick up stuff earlier and treat easier. But from my age etc he thinks the genetic stuff is unlikely...so feel a LOT more positive now x*
>
> *He was also saying that I really surprised him in getting out of hospital within 48 hrs… as it just doesn't happen… and he was fully expecting me to stay in 7 days! He was pleased I have healed really well. And he laughed was I back to normal- but still not 'normal' – as i agreed, that would be an insult! ☺*
>
> *I truly think the homeopathy helped, and also the power of healing from others and me asking Angels … as I know that*

deep down , once I heard I made it through the op and all was well and saw the shadow figures by my bed , I knew I was safe.
I just need to keep remembering that. ♥

It was odd, as he said that I really should be 'proud' of myself (I agreed I had lived my nightmare and survived...just before I burst into tears on him!) ...and stop sweating the small stuff. And he seems very much Mr Conventional Surgeon! Although he did listen to me saying they need ginger tea, manuka honey and arnica for all patients in hospital... (although maybe he didn't have much choice on listening to that! ☺)

But the best bit is that my head is finally feeling more normal ☺ I had two cranial sessions and while it felt super tight immediately after, it is now feeling far better. Still numb when I touch, but when I don't it mostly feels ok x

A funny old lesson this one..."

24th August. Posted on Facebook.

"I have a tufty bit of hair ☺ ♥
Good job I cannot see the back ☺"

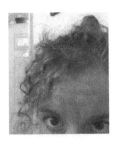

At the end of August I try and go into the Kingston Vodafone store to ask them can I get a low SAR phone. The staff there have absolutely no idea what I am talking about, attempt to look up SAR ratings on their system but say they have no details about the ratings and I will just have to check each phone. The guy talks to someone else and they say they think the new Samsung phones are lower than many, but I look at the phones and they are stupid money. I am not paying even £100 for a phone I am barely going to use, much less £400-£600! Believe me, when you have had a brain tumour and you still have two holes in your skull you don't want to put any mobile device emitting EMFs anywhere near your head. I tell the staff this and the guy just looks blankly at me. Surely someone working at a mobile phone shop would know there are links to mobile phone use and brain tumours... or maybe they just don't want to consider the thought when their job revolves around it?

After a few days (I am still a bit slow doing everything) I call the Vodafone helpline (on the landline) and tell them I want to cancel my contract, and the 3 staff that I speak to online in my attempt to cancel it all ask me why I am cancelling. I say as I had a brain tumour and I don't want to use a mobile except for emergencies anymore, yet none of the people I speak to seem to give a shit. I am so annoyed with their attitude that I change to a pay as you go phone where I can call others on the same network for free. (I was paying for this with Vodafone)

I look online and find there is a really low SAR phone called a Doro that I can buy on E-bay for about £60 from a store where it is new, but the box has been opened. And to top it it's simple and supposedly built for older people with bigger buttons on the touchscreen. Result. Especially when your coordination is still not the best!

I also have ordered a Vitali-Chi machine a week or so ago, it arrives along with the remedies specifically designed for me. So each day I try and use it for about 40 minutes. It is great as I am still needing to rest each day and so this makes me calm down and meditate, with the added bonus that I feel deeply relaxed while I am using it, but also more invigorated once I have finished. Almost every time I use it, I fall soundly asleep and then wake up just before the last of the meditation songs stops. It is really odd as the area where the tumour was physically tingles while I am using the machine, but it feels good tingling, like it is helping me heal.

26th August. Calla has her enrolment day for starting college, Dave drops us both off in the car outside the college. It feels the first time in a very long time that I am actually doing anything useful for my kids. I am being a normal mum again.

Although I also have to explain to the tutors (whom I know, and had already told I was having a brain tumour removed, as Zach has just finished this exact same course) that she only got a D in Maths when she needs a C to not have to re-sit it at college. I explain that I didn't realise until a couple of weeks ago I could apply for 'special consideration' to gain an extra 5% on her marks, which would be enough to give her a C, due to the fact she was home educated (and I couldn't educate her at all this year) and she took her exams while I was in hospital.

Really I know it was not my fault that she failed to get a C in the exams she took this year, I didn't ask to be ill while she was working towards her exams this year, nor have brain tumour surgery in the middle of her exams… but I still feel awful and somehow responsible that I have affected her, even if I know that after college her exam results will not even be relevant.

2nd September. Posted to a friend.

"Mercury in retrograde must be getting to me or something... ☹
I need ideas...
I feel deep inside that I need to move. Yes there is the physical stuff (surburbia pollution etc) but it is far more than that... it's just a massive urge to have somewhere natural (or more natural than here!) to live... I have wanted to do something for ages, the 'Anastasia' books where you have your own kin garden just fill me with love and longing, as do cob houses... I have said to Dave 14 or so years ago that I wanted to move, but held on here for the kids at school, then college etc so as not to disrupt them...
...then yesterday eldest said something that really made me think...I have done this for years for them and Dave, but now I HAVE to do what I want for me.
Tried to explain to Dave but he just doesn't get that deep inside I NEED to do something, he just keeps saying, louder and louder 'give me your reasons' like they are all logical or something and I am not explaining them. (I can't even drive and fuck off properly which I so wanted to!)

I also have been struggling with saying words at times since before op and so he doesn't get the frustration that putting me under stress means I just cannot find the words even more... and I can't explain it's a deep gut feeling. Even though I am happy he follows his passions as much as he can and I accept that. (our lives revolve around his bands and music)

I am looking for possible house swaps... but so far no one wants to come here where I would also want to go to (let alone kids or Dave) ... and I can't even get them to really agree on areas or even look. Calla is also at a local college this year, Zach is starting at Guildford ACM for a music degree course commuting from here, but if we moved could no doubt find accommodation. Adam is needing to get his own place after university (though currently in my art shed ☹) & we still have Roan in our bedroom (he's 10 soon!) ... 3 bedrooms with 6 people (and girlfriends!) doesn't work...

I have thought of getting a static caravan somewhere southwards so I can escape at times, but then all I can see is a ground rent that I can nowhere near afford, and that's not even starting on the caravan price, and I probably can't grow veggies etc.

Dave's Dad has the caravan in Norfolk, but its 3 hours' drive away and not even near public transport (we have 1 car and I can't even drive for another 3 months or so.. not that I have much energy either) and then it's not 'mine'..

Am I missing any other possibilities?? Northwards is cheaper, but less warm and I struggle with the lack of sun as it is! I have no money, no income, and no passion atm. I am still struggling with my eyesight and even colouring in books ... let alone art. Unless i go truly abstract?! But i just don't want to do it and fail... and no idea on how to get enough money from it even if my health was totally ok. My energy is still lower than before op, and i still feel I'm recovering... emotionally for sure ☹

...and the weather is getting colder ☹"

24th September. Posted on Facebook.

"Fuck...just found this: "Frustrations of a Brain Surgeon" (1)

...same hospital, same wards, same surgeon...think it's the same area of head (though different type of tumour) ...

but hey...i was out of there in 2 days ❤ ... and they had spare beds at the time (they even shut the special care ward down for a while after I left)
but fuck! ❤ (actually maybe the fuck comments were why they sent me home? ☺)"

Then later on:

"Having to fill in forms to get driving licence back, and have to include consultants details...but it's a bit odd when I go on the St George's website and get a smiling face of the guy who basically saved my life (he said the number of consultants who will have operated on my blood vessel tumour are limited!)
Thanks, Mr Jones! ❤
(although looking up his details now is not anywhere near as bad as having to do so before I had the surgery!- it's still pretty emotional ❤)"

It might sound odd to most people, but having to sort these forms and fill my paperwork is really tough. It's confusing to have to find all the details and I feel I am struggling with it, and writing the details in is still quite hard to do and make the writing legible. I especially struggle with having to fill the forms out in block capital letters as I do not seem to be able to control the pen correctly. I just cannot concentrate properly and if I have to do so I just get really tearful and annoyed with myself that my ability is so poor. I hope this gets better with time. I am also wanting to send an official complaint letter about my (lack of) diagnosis to my G.P surgery, but now it all takes so much time. I feel I need to get things correct, and yet doing so means it takes me far longer to remember things (I need to make notes for weeks before even attempting to write anything) and trying to word it all in sensible date order and just make sure it reads clearly is hard. It is things I know- yet it feels so hard, like I am writing an assignment where I have to include medical facts and references in a subject I know nothing about. Plus I have the interesting problem of constantly typing words wrong, so instead of surgery I write sugrery and with that I am constantly pressing back and rewriting words. I also seem to have lost my ability to spell and have to think each sound and therefore letter out on many longer words that I knew quite easily before. As well part of my coordination as to where the letters are on the keyboard seems to be missing, so I need to be able to see each individual letter on the keyboard clearly too! It takes me so long to even write a few paragraphs. But hey, at least I can see the screen now without it spinning and actually type - even if it is slow.

28th September. Posted on Facebook a photo of this text from a book I am reading.

From The Brain's Way of Healing. By Norman Doidge.
"Elizabeth Natenshon, whom I interviewed, was born missing a third of her cerebellum, a part of the brain that helps to coordinate and control the timing of movement, thought, balance and attention. Without the cerebellum, a person has difficulty controlling all these mental functions. The cerebellum, which means 'little brain' in Latin, is about the size of a peach and is tucked under the cerebral hemispheres, towards the back of the brain. Although it occupies only about 10 percent of the brain's volume, it contains almost 80 percent of the brain's neurons."

"Interesting that this brain healing book says the cerebellum is related to movement, thought, balance and attention... As I feel it had been despite what anyone has said – and that its just balance and coordination!
But if this girl with a third her cerebellum missing (where

Dr's said she would be severely retarded at best) can get 2
degrees, get married & and be normal ... I've got no fucking
excuse ♥ *"*

10th October. It feels it has taken weeks to get my head around
writing a complaint to the G.P surgery – a mixture of events that are
serious and need to be comprehensive and factually correct. I have
written down ideas, and then added in the detail. Having to leave
things a few weeks to see if I remember anything else and also give
myself time so I don't get too stressed in writing this. Finally today
the complaint letter has gone in the post.

11th October. I ask on Facebook.

> *"My hair is annoying me...*
> *I still feel like I have a wig in parts of my head at the back as*
> *it's so numb (and so keep pulling it and don't know) and*
> *can't manage hairclips or even bands anywhere near where*
> *it still feels odd (they dig in and feel awful) and obviously*
> *have some interesting tufty bits that are growing back at*
> *both the front and back.*
> *...so for the first time in years I am thinking of getting a*
> *decent haircut. Any ideas on what style or shall I just surprise*
> *you all (and myself!)??"*

14th October. I decide I am going to get my hair cut. I don't want to
in many ways, but also I feel that if I get the length cut off and so
stop pulling it when I don't realise and getting a numb head feeling
as a result; that by the time it grows back I will either have more
feeling again or will be able to cope with it better, and I won't need
any hair clips that feel they stick into my head. Plus I have short bits
of hair throughout – if the rest is cut shorter it won't be so obvious.

So I sit at the hairdressers and ask him to cut it about shoulder length, with the back slightly shorter than the front to compensate for the short areas while still leaving it look as long as possible (and so the back is all the correct hairstyle length all over and not with any shorter parts from the shaved areas during the operation). I am simultaneously happy to have it cut shorter (for the first time since I was about 13!) and see what it looks like and yet it also feels like I have lost a part of me too. A sacrifice I didn't and still don't want to make. My Nan's voice is inside my head telling me that she hopes I will never need my red curls cut for a brain tumour...

Chapter 27 - Positively Negative

15th October. I go out again for another gig with Dave and on the bar of the pub see a charity tin for 'The Brain Tumour Charity'. I write the name of the website down on my phone – I know I won't remember it otherwise.

The next morning I look at their website and actually find both information on hemangioblastoma and information about what issues tumours in the cerebellum can cause. *"If a brain tumour is located in the cerebellum, symptoms may include difficulty with: Balance, A loss of co-ordination, Difficulty walking and speaking, Flickering of the eyes, Vomiting, Stiff neck, Problems with dexterity. (skills in using your hands)"*

Wow! Of these I had all but vomiting (although had nausea) and told them to the G.P on more than one occasion.

Plus it says: *"Headaches associated with brain tumours are usually severe, throbbing, worse in the morning (you may wake with one) and aggravated by straining or coughing."* What? Aggravated by straining and coughing is a 'sign' of brain tumours?! I am fucking livid!! As apart from the first locum G.P. I definitely told each of the doctor's I saw this was happening as I <u>knew</u> it was significant. (And this was the phrase I was searching online when I came up with Chiari malformation) How did it not ring any alarm bells to supposedly trained medical professionals? Plus I know I even asked all three doctors 'could it be a brain tumour?' – as I knew that waking with headaches, or having them at night was a symptom, so it's not like the thought of a brain tumour wasn't mentioned to them either. But with all these signs, how did they not see it staring them in the face?? It is <u>so</u> damn obvious to me now. It just seems they dismissed it, but how can someone who's very job is to recognise these type of symptoms manage to miss it? Just how?

18th October. I finally receive a letter back from the genetics clinic saying:

> *"I am pleased to inform you that no mutation was identified in the VHL gene. This makes it very unlikely that you have a diagnosis of Von Hippel-Lindau syndrome as you have no other features of the condition... although it is very unlikely that you have the diagnosis of VHL, we like to follow up all patients with isolated cerebellar haemangioblastoma until the age of 60 years on a two yearly basis..."*

Yes, Yes, YES!!!! My kids won't get this. This is all that really matters...

24th October. Written to friend.

> *"Just to say I got a letter to say that they don't think tumour was from the VHL genetic cause ... All tests negative ☺ ♥ ♥ Am still due 2 yearly scans (the genetics team now won't do head MRI – that stays with neuro team) but I don't have the possibility that the kids each have a 50% risk of the same ♥ ♥ ♥ ♥ ♥*
> *I think I can deal with my stuff better now... Xx"*

12th November. Written to friend.

"I know it's getting near full moon again (and all my issues always get worse) but I just want to cry at someone who will listen …

Dave says – without listening- to my tears that I should shut up and tells me I am driving myself mental ☹ but sometimes I just struggle with the after effects since my op and want to talk about the huge emotions it brings up …

My front scar is getting so deep it is again freaking me if I touch it, but it itches … The back scar area is just numb to touch still and if I lean on my head wrong it just goes worse and feels numb all over … I have what feels like a really sore patch of ripped hair (not near either scar) on the top of my head and my neck muscles are screwed … I know my body is still not central.

I SO get that I'm alive still and know how terrified I was and that I survived it… But I feel it's still up in the air.

I am still waiting to drive, but am scared of doing so again and being by myself. Scared that I have my 6 month MRI soon and what it will show … Terrified actually.

I want to talk to a support group, nurse or something … But I cannot find who. The G.P's are fucking useless, the surgeon's secretary says they will get back to me after MRI if I need more follow up, and there is no nurse etc. There was a support group (for benign tumours) but I cannot see that it's still running and get no answer from email. The online brain tumour support groups are full of people with brain cancer and that is just too much to cope with …after all they would love my result! And so I feel a fraud for complaining!!!

I need reassurance but can't find it... So just have to look inwards ... At times I can feel the strength and love of something far bigger than me (and often shivers up my spine) and then sometimes I just crack ... (I want the external support ... ☹) Something reminds me how close I was to not still being here and I just open floods of tears ....

I'm in one of those now.

This year has been tough and I'm mentally exhausted ☹

(Also have been doing my complaint letter to G.P and everything still takes me longer than before ... It's so slow !)"

13th November. Posted on Facebook.

"Just realised I can type in the dark again (I'm on laptop.) ♥ My coordination must be returning as I haven't been able to do this for months! ☺ ♥ "

This might be a short post, and seemingly minor to most people, but to be able to type even frequent words without having to look at each and every letter is amazing. To be able to type a sentence in the dark when I cannot see each letter also gives me back another part of me. I have not been able to do this since about February.

14th November. At my neuro-physiotherapist appointment today, I tell them that I have started to do the 'moving my head from side to side' exercises while I am walking the dog at the park. I look at either the dog or a fixed object and walk along turning my head from side to side, or tipping it up and down. It feels like it is helping me more doing it this way than standing somewhere marching on the spot, and as I walk Enzo every day it's a good practice to do and

I can repeat it several times over with each walk. She agrees that this will be great way to practice this. I also say I often walk along the marked lines of the football pitch and as I am doing so shut my eyes for a few seconds to see how far I veer off course. Normally after just a few steps I am about a foot to one side of the line, but I don't feel anywhere near as wobbly as I did a few weeks ago when I first started trying this. She tells me that she can see the difference already.

I sometimes wonder what anyone walking past thinks off this woman seemingly either nodding or shaking her head as she is walking around with her dog, what they have judged me as. If they are that small minded to have judged me negatively- then I wouldn't want to speak to them anyway and, if I am honest, I actually don't care anymore. Plus I have the benefit of walking around doing odd things might keep people away- I actually quite like my walk in silence and being able to cry when I need to, it's quite therapeutic and healing.

18th November.

> *"6 months ago I was about to walk down the corridor at St Georges to the operating theatre … Shaking so much they had to give me a heated air cushion to warm myself up in there!!*
> *Today I have a haircut, a numb head and some rather large scars hidden in my hair …. But I'm here* ❤
> *I probably still look the same on the outside but the inside is oh so different now* ❤
> *Thanks for putting up with me* ☺"

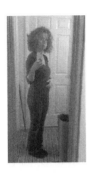

Today is also 6 months after my operation, the date I was told I would be able to get my driving licence back and it also says 6 months after the surgery on the DVLA forms and their website, yet I have no driving licence. I have done the vision tests at the opticians that they asked and the optometrist said all was ok. I call DVLA to find out what is happening and get told that they have all the correct paperwork and surgeon's letter, but they are processing my details and it will take a few more weeks. Fucking great. I applied 6 weeks before my licence was due back- the maximum time they say to apply and they still haven't done it! Maybe they should let you apply a little earlier than this if they cannot process things in this time? Good job I am not trying to use my licence to go back to work.

22nd November. Today is follow up MRI day. I feel a little scared and nauseous. What if they find the tumour has not been fully removed or is growing back already? What if they see another hemangioblastoma in my body somewhere? I somehow feel that this is the real result day.

So again I get to the hospital feeling a little nervous, and Dave and I sit in the radiology waiting room while I am fidgeting. It seems to be that today they are running late with the MRI, which isn't helping my stress levels much. Eventually I am called down to the room outside the scanner and asked to change into a gown, but I say I don't wear wired bras, haven't got any metal clips and purposely just have t-shirt material on today, so they tell me I am ok as I am and to just wait a little while they prepare the scanner. I give them my meditation CD I have brought to play while they scan me.

They call me in and I ask did they want to give me the contrast dye (gadolinium) with this scan? They reply that yes they do. I tell them I am not happy having this routinely as it's a toxic heavy metal and could they please do the MRI without it. I don't know if no one normally refuses to have this, but I feel I am being awkward and get asked what am I being scanned for? "A brain tumour". Then I am told that the contrast helps to see if there are any small areas left over or re-growing and so I say I know there is that risk, but 'if' there is anything that is so small they cannot see it on the MRI without the contrast, then I don't want to know anyway, and I don't want the contrast injected in my body without very good reason. They tell me that's a fair point, as long as I understand and have reasons, and so I say thank you and get in the machine.

I don't think this MRI scanner is as modern as the private MRI scan I had last time, or at least it doesn't feel it. It doesn't feel as comfortable and the headrest and what goes over you doesn't seem to be as simple for the staff to put me in, but this time the noise is awful. With my previous one there were only a few instances where I couldn't hear my CD and it seemed it was only as they were doing the last few seconds on each area, this time it seemed that most of the time the noises from the machine covered up the CD. There was one song that was about 10 minutes long that I think I only heard two short bursts of! And yes the CD when I could hear it was about as loud as it was last time.

I am guessing after 20 or so minutes I am getting a head pain in the left side of my head, it's grinding into the centre of my head and I am really trying to keep listening to my meditation. Imagining the meditation when I cannot hear a thing. I want to move position – maybe laying on this plastic surface is digging into my head? But know I have to keep still as the stiller I am the quicker this will be done, so again I go back to silently praying to angels to keep me calm, stop the pain, make the results great and send the universe love. I ignore the feeling in my head and focus on love and strength instead, that power that got me out of hospital after 48 hours. If I can do brain surgery, I can do this for several more hours without moving a millimetre. I trust. I trust I am ok. I focus on the feeling in the rest of my body and I swear they scanned down my spine in levels, first near my neck, then nearer the middle of my spine - down until my hip area. As every so often it felt that a different area was heating up and I could feel the pulse of the machine below it. The voice then comes over my earphones and they tell me they have scanned it all. I get out of the machine and even while I am in the same room, the head pain that's been there for the last 30 minutes or so instantly disappears. We go home. And now we wait...

Chapter 28 - All in One Song

28 November. Posted on Facebook.

"Today's message... Please don't judge on appearances. I was actually pushed in the back to move me out of the way this eve – when leaning on the bar when I was trying to video Dave's band in a pub. I was there as I didn't want anyone dancing nearby to hit the back of my head as it still feels delicate after brain surgery and has a plate in it and the fact that my balance still isn't perfect and I felt I needed support to lean on for a bit.

I was not drunk, I don't drink, yet this is twice this has happened this year ☹

Yes everyone says I look really well now, but I have spent 6 months solid feeling totally drunk and off balance this year due to a tumour in my cerebellum. Even sitting down I was spinning at times and I know I walked into people as well as things! ☹ *The tumour was only removed 6 mths ago and I still have neuro physio sessions. Thankfully it was removed* ❤ *but many people who look well are still affected with balance or health conditions.*

If you want me to move (even if there was a gap when I got there) please ask. ❤

But don't judge or push... You don't know what health issues someone may have or what's going on inside.

And if you think it's still ok to push someone out of your way then I suggest you seek counselling ...

And yes I did politely tell you after the song finished why I found it offensive ... And you just looked rudely back at me! ☹

Hopefully you will think twice if it happens again? ❤ *"*

6th December. I have an appointment with a standard physiotherapist in regard to my neck muscles having such a dip in them on my right side. When I get there she asks what surgery I have had done, and then when she feels the muscle, asks if any of my muscles were removed. I have no idea. I never thought about this being a possibility, but as she says it I think and tell her "I am missing a part of my skull, so 'if' they were attached to that part then maybe they would no longer be there, but I don't know". I get given a few exercises that may help build them up, but she tells me they will only work if there are muscles there to build up. Oh why don't I even know what happened to me? It's so hard to deal with not knowing...

8th December. Calla and I decide to go pottery painting. I want to just paint and relax as much as I need to see if my control and vision have got better. When we get there I feel I should paint a 'splat' bowl, so paint it in several base colours and then decorate over it with simple bold patterns and dots. I still cannot concentrate on the same area for too long, my eyes just don't seem to manage it, but its far better than it was. Somewhere in the middle of painting, and realising I am able to do this for a short time without hardly any problem, even if it is simple, and I feel the need to write the word 'TRUST' on the inside of the bowl. It's back to that word. I just need to trust that I will be able to heal and do things I want again in time.

9th December. I am getting impatient. Why have I not heard anything re my MRI yet? So I ask Dave to call Mr Jones' secretary to find out when we will get the result. His secretary says that there would have been a radiographer looking at the MRI as they scanned me, so if there was anything serious she would have been told instantly and we would most certainly have been contacted by now, so not to worry. She also confirms with Dave that they sent the paperwork off to the DVLA ages ago, without any concerns.

Written to friend.

*"Am still having to go with the 'no news is good news' as still
no definite results since my MRI – now well over 2 weeks ago
(they said I should know within 10 days) but Dave called
surgeon's secretary today and she said anything serious
would have been seen as they did the scan and so they/we
would have been told by now. So it's good i guess! But I just
so want confirmation that there is nothing of the tumour left
in my skull and it's not growing back...*

*I also have not been able to see surgeon re the side effects or
even get a reply to my email questions... I have not seen
anyone since August. The G.P. knew nothing, neuro-
physiotherapist neither... even DVLA seems to just be
processing my driving licence – and in no rush!*

...so I'm waiting a bit more!!

*I guess I just want to know if the feelings in my head since
are all normal, (I know surgeon said I would always have
side effects...but be alive...   )*

*... and I guess I have to accept I will never know the 'cause'...
and in fact thinking unconventionally makes it all even more
confusing!"*

10th December. Today I receive this letter in the post

*"I have seen your scan from this week and all looks excellent
with no residual tumour. I am very happy with your progress
and as I understand that the team will be following you up
with regular scans and so forth in due course. If there are
any problems in the future do drop me a line.*

With many thanks

Yours sincerely

Mr Timothy Jones. Consultant Neurosurgeon"

"YEAH!!!" ♥ ♥ ♥ Finally! I guess my brain is OK and there are no signs of anything else in my spine. Does that mean this nightmare is all but over? Hopefully my emotions will be able to catch up soon and let this all be just history.

12/12/16. Posted on Facebook.

> "AND discharged from neuro physio today I even got 29 out of 30! ♥ Not bad for someone that couldn't put even one foot in front of the other (drink drive testing style) from Jan-May ...now I can manage a room length! ☺

As I look at my Neuro-physio appointments card today, I realise that the appointments were on 9/9/16, 10/10/16, 12/12/16 – and I said I was getting lots of doubled numbers when I really felt I needed some strength and support.

18th December 2016

> "So for today's little rambling of the darkest days of the year... ☺
>
> Last night I was watching Dave play ... they were playing Freebird at the time... And suddenly I was sitting there (alone) singing along from what suddenly felt like the core of me and the emotions from the past year came up and I just continued singing the rest with tears of every emotion running down my face...
>
> I had been to the local Buddhist temple earlier and they were talking about how peoples' response can vary due to their life at the time... And how if you were driving and thanked someone they might not acknowledge you at that time due to circumstances that were nothing to do with you.

And suddenly the feelings of May came back... of knowing I had a fucking brain tumour... They were going to have to open MY head up soon ... There was a good chance I would need a blood transfusion... The chance of a stroke or something negative... The surgeon saying I might hate him after.... I might bleed to death... This might be it... Having felt dizzy (or as I remember the feeling of being drunk) for 4-5 months - solidly...not able to walk and touch one foot in front if the other...unable to turn my head without pain...exhausted from the fight or flight that hit me each time I wobbled (many times a day) and the pain of nightly headaches. I couldn't turn to look to cross roads ... Dave had to hold me each time ... Or even to walk ... Knowing that to live I had no choice but to have this op... To totally trust...

And I was being driven to hospital to go and get my increased headache checked - still not due the op for another 9 days (but what ended up being the day I went to hospital before op as they kept me in) ... And every single thing driving there was painful... Every red light... Every person crossing in front of us... Each person who pulled out...

And comparing it to going home after the op... I was leaving the hospital 48 hours after I came out of theatre (when I was told I would be there 5-9 days or possibly more... And I would <u>not</u> be able to leave earlier!) ... I hadn't needed a blood transfusion ... I was able to touch my feet together when I walked ... The neck pain had gone (although huge swelling and cut neck muscles replaced it) ... But I was alive!!!! And going home ... Going home to be able to cuddle my 'babies' (even if the youngest was 9) Tell them that it was going to be ok now... And not see the terrified look on their faces ... It didn't matter that I had 40 staples in my head... That I looked like I felt- and hadn't slept properly for weeks! ... But this time even shitty parts of Tooting seemed amazing - like really seeing it for the first time as a tourist would ...

Who cares if a car pulled out in front... Their day job might have been shit ... They can't help it they are stuck in the rat race... This thing most of us call life... They need the love and understanding - not me! We could just let them and their rushing or even aggressiveness go... I was going home and it didn't matter if it took 1.5 hours....

And so last night I experienced all these feelings -and more - in a few minutes... In one song ... watching couples hug and dance with each other...

And it reminded me just how blessed we all are to be alive...
"

There is no choice
You die or be brave
But you are scared
...so very scared

Yet you have to let go
Release the fears
Trust
Trust in others
Trust in a higher power
And release

The universe has your back
You're still alive
And you're free
...so very free.

Chapter 29 - A New Year

A week or so before Christmas I call DVLA up and ask has my driving licence been processed yet, and they tell me it is still being sorted. I half shout and half cry at them saying this is ridiculous, you said I would not have my licence for 6 months only. I applied for it when you stated to on your website, I haven't had any issues and the surgeon has sent you paperwork weeks ago and yet you still have not processed it. Now it's Christmas and my husband will still have to drive everywhere as I am not able to and I should have got my licence back over a month ago. It's so frustrating. The woman sort of apologises and says they have a backlog but it is being done, so I sort of hang up saying 'please sort it' at the same time.

Although in some ways I am a little relieved. I have no pressure of 'having' to drive when I feel tired, or when others want me to taxi them around when they have had a drink. I can't. I don't have a driving licence.

1st January 2017. Written in journal.

> "So it has taken me this long to put pen to paper again. I'm not sure if it's laziness or fear of crying a river if I truly feel the magnitude of emotions I have now and have felt over the past few months.
>
> But I think I have had to shut part of me away, for I wasn't ready to cope with it.
> Only today, 7 ½ months after my operation have I dared look online at where the muscles, nerves and skull actually are in your head. I wasn't able to look and deal with it before. And now I know – there is basically one big nerve running up the back on each side of your head. And mines been cut…

I didn't realise this before or just after the operation (I'm not blaming the surgeon – he probably told me. I just didn't listen. I wasn't ready.) Only the day after the op did I realise they cut my neck muscles to get in my skull! (Ahh! That explains the huge neck pain and swelling!)

Yet I still thought the numbness up the sides and top of my head was an after effect of the op, but that it would go with the swelling. Damaged tissue or something.
But when I went back at 3 weeks he told me that the main nerve was cut. I would always have a numb patch, although the other nerves would try and compensate in time.

I know I should be grateful it is one of the worst side effects, but it was totally a bolt inside when he told me. I didn't realise before, but I would never feel my head properly again!

It sounds stupid, but I had to mourn it. I was in shock. As he said it and the reality sank in, once again I was trying not to just be a blubbering wreck. I could feel my eyes welling up and I just had to bite my lip and not express the enormity of my emotions. But even as I was hiding the tears I also knew that I was so thankful for what I still had (The tumour had gone. I was OK) and not what I hadn't now got. And the enormity of that gratitude also hit me at the same time, and so I wanted to cry tears of joy too!

And now…if I shut my eyes and relax now… I am still Jo. I can shut my eyes and still feel the same bliss inside, or I can feel pain. Sometimes the pain wins, sometimes the bliss.

Sometimes I feel it's a circle of feelings:
Itching – what feels like it is under my skull and I cannot scratch it.

Tenderness – where I feel like I have a bruise near where the plate must be. Numbness – that if I lean on the 'wrong part' it feels like my whole right side of my head has an ½ cm thick layer of papier-mâché on it, it all moves and 'digs in' as one plate. Catching my hair makes it feel like this.
Nerve pain – where it feels like my hair has been ripped out and is sore.
Itchy scar at front – but the scar is too deep that I can't touch it"

On the first work day in January I call the DVLA up, and start to let rip as to where my driving licence is, just as the woman tells me it went in the post this morning so I can legally drive now as it is on all the records as it has already been given. I stutter and ask why it took seven and a half months and not six, and she says sorry we have been really backlogged. But finally I have it. I can drive again!

8.1.17. Written in journal.

"Not sure exactly what I want to write, but I just feel SO emotional. Like I could cry a river from all the emotions I feel right now, over the past year.

I don't think its sadness – just enormous gratitude, relief, letting go of the fear, exhaustion (physical and mental), love, tinged with a bit of frustration as to why the world can be so evil and why others can't see this way...

I finally got my driving licence back, hence I managed to go to FMG. (The group is energetically based on the pioneering work of 'The Journey' by Brandon Bays and on the power of stillness for deep personal and spiritual transformation.) *I haven't been able to go for a whole year and longed just to be allowed to 'be'. Laugh, cry – whatever – it's all OK! To be with others who 'get it, get that emotions are OK and try to build spirituality into their lives.*

It feels like I have sobbed since I let the floodgates open there. I still have so much I need to release.

Saying I had brain surgery still feels like it happened to someone else, but I have this fuck off great scar on my head, a hole at the front and numbness to remind me. Daily. Hourly. Every few minutes.

But the really, really odd thing is... that despite all those crap feelings, the lack of being able to discuss it, the whole experience when looked at as 'one' has been positive.

Or as the quote on Facebook said the other day...

'This year has been both the worst and best year of my life.'

It actually seems a little mad saying it's the best year – but I was given another chance of life. And that's got to be celebrated!!

Thing is, as totally terrified and scared that I was – I never thought that I was dying. Maybe I was and people never think that they are? Or maybe, deep down, I just knew it wasn't my time? My fear took over at times – yes. I was so scared of what could go wrong. Numb from the shock. Had panic attacks so constantly that it seemed like they were normal days.

But after the op, that I knew I had survived it and had my angelic shadows in the room. I know there is something bigger than me, or what humans see on earth. We get support. There is a bigger plan."

Maybe Rudolf Steiner was right when he said that age 42 was the start of your spiritual growth?!

Chapter 30 - The Hole in my Head

19th January 2017. I am now on the third official complaint letter to the G.P surgery. It is madness. I do get they don't want to admit they did anything wrong as that would mean they would need to compensate me. But they fucked up, they fucked up big time. Not once, but on several appointments, I gave (what I now know are) signs and symptoms of a brain tumour and fluid on my brain, yet they didn't even refer me and the doctors actually said a brain tumour would be very unlikely. Plus it is pretty poor management that after failing to diagnose me they also did not check my 'urgent' neurosurgery referral letter was sent off, as well as failing to remove my staples after the operation. They even admitted they had a 'significant event analysis meeting' after they realised I had a brain tumour- surely that in itself is acknowledgement that they know they could have done things better?

But the letters are just so stupid. Do they really think that I would expect a G.P to write on her notes that 'she rolled her eyes at me', or that she was thinking I am just a little neurotic and so offered me diazepam rather than send me for an MRI or the neurologist that I requested? Of course they wouldn't, but it doesn't mean they didn't think it. Just because the notes 'aren't there' doesn't mean it didn't happen. The letter was so ridiculous and didn't answer any of my questions properly, that I basically rewrite my last letter but this time highlight the questions I want answered in yellow and add extra 'these are simple questions I want answered' written in red alongside it.

I am the one who has just dealt with a brain tumour and am struggling at times to think and write, yet their letters are like they had a school child on a work experience day write what they thought and no one bothered to check it before posting. It's all just waffle and no substance. As they say "bullshit baffles brains"... or stops you responding as it all takes so much effort.

20th January. A lovely practitioner and friend Marion suggests I do some 'Journey Work' with her. (Based on Brandon Bays book – the Journey) So I go to 'The Sanctuary', a lovely old church in Ewell that has been converted into a holistic venue where you can feel the calm radiating from the walls. I go deep into relaxation and feel what I am saying is helpful and enlightening, sometimes a little tearful, but calm. Then a really odd thing happens, just as Marion says to 'imagine the messages being sent in by the Angels and God going into the crown of my head', I start laughing! Suddenly I find it more than slightly amusing and sit there with my eyes shut and the biggest, silliest grin on my face saying to Marion. "I don't need them to send anything through my crown, I already have a hole, a direct portal into my brain. I now know if they want me to."

Marion continues calmly saying to feel where the messages are going in, and suddenly I can touch this deep hole at the top of my head, really put my fingers onto it and feel the dent and it is ok. It's truly ok. I am still laughing at it and say to her "I couldn't touch it before, it was too deep and made me feel a bit sick, but now it's fine, it's my portal for when I need to listen to something, to understand something. As I touch it now, I can feel the love that healed me..." and yet again I am sitting crying, but this time with tears of joy.

This is the summary of the messages that Marion wrote down for me:

You are here to wake people up.

Your biggest resource is trust.

Whether things are good or bad depends on how you view them.
(Your thoughts are all that matters)

Let 'positive emotions' trickle into your body (so you can slowly absorb them) 'they' know you've got it already.

You don't need to rush.

We're here, just ask. (Angels)

Angels need to be part of your book

I go home, and for the first time in a long while I truly feel at peace. I know I have tapped into emotions that I have never really felt before, I understand them. I've known before that I should feel this way, but it wasn't really 'in there'. Now it feels like it is starting, I don't need to rush, just let the emotions trickle in and it will all be as I need it. I can trust it's all ok

23rd January. Written to Marion today.

> *"Thank you once again for the Journey work on Friday, I am still totally fine with touching my hole in my head -in fact it feels a hole showing my strength and inner power, and know I need to continue with what I am doing (even if others, or outside says it's not enough) and continue to write the book– albeit slowly!*
>
> *Someone was talking with me about my head and operation on Saturday and I was much calmer and had the feeling that it was ok and what was meant to be... and also distanced now. Not so raw and painful.*
> *So thank you again ❤"*

31st January. I get another letter back from G.P surgery, this time with completely the wrong details on it… amongst a few other concerns, their letter clearly states that Dr Vo ONLY offered me diazepam as she saw on the neck x-ray that my muscles were twisted and so diazepam would help relax them. Fair point. IF she hadn't sent me to get my neck x-rayed AFTER I saw her!! (and I had written all the dates in my complaint letters)… Can I scream at how incompetent they are? This is supposedly their reply to my official complaint and they get the details totally wrong and so can't even come up with a vaguely valid reason why I was offered diazepam! Muscle spasm was clearly a valid reason…but IF she had asked me to have the x-ray at this point. I hadn't, so obviously this wasn't why she offered it to me. How can anyone that is supposed to be caring for your health get even this basic information and the dates so wrong?

That's it. I am not even going to bother to reply, they have the details of the health ombudsman on their letter saying to contact them if I am not happy with their answer, so I will now be writing to them instead. And changing G.P surgery. I have lost all confidence that the doctors at Giggs Hill know anything.

It takes me about 2 weeks to process the information, copy out all the letters I have sent and received back from the G.P and write a covering letter to the health ombudsman to complain.

16th February.

> "Finally written to health ombudsman about shite treatment from GPs last year. Huge envelope to go in post!
> Gave up with G.P's reply- they can't even get the basic facts right telling me one GP offered me valium due to my x-ray result- when she was the one that sent me there AFTER her appointment!!!

And they won't admit any wrongdoing even though they had a 'significant events meeting' over my case as to how they could have done better in diagnosing me...um...surely that means they know they fucked up?!"

18th February. So I might have been right all along? I said from before I knew I had a tumour that I knew my 'fight or flight' reflexes were going a little into overdrive, and that I assumed it was just as when I started to fall or wobble that was the result, but today I see this article which basically says:

"For the first time, neuroscientists at University of Bristol have identified a brain pathway that may be the root of the universal response to freeze in place when we are afraid. Their revolutionary study—released on April 23, 2014— discovered a chain of neural connections stemming from the cerebellum.
These new discoveries on the neurobiology of fear responses are a first step toward better understanding the role that the cerebellum might be playing in the paralyzing power of anxiety, phobias, and fear in general." (2)

So as the whole area of my cerebellum either had a tumour pushing into it, or lots of swelling and extra fluid, no wonder I felt I was going insane. Somehow this helps me make a little more sense of what I had been feeling. And maybe gives me the prospect that once the area has fully healed and settled I will be able to relax a little more.

20th February. Shared and posted on Facebook an article about 'Preventing and Healing Brain Tumours'... some of which says:

"Practicing stress reduction techniques such as yoga, meditation, and breathing exercises can reduce stress. While practicing these techniques, inhaling frankincense oil can help alleviate inflammation in the brain.

One of the major causes of death related to brain tumors is inflammation from swelling in the brain. When frankincense extract was administered to patients before surgery they experienced reduced swelling and fluid accumulation during and after treatment. Patients also exhibited fewer symptoms of brain damage.

Boswellic acid is the main active component found in frankincense traditionally used to treat arthritis, asthma, and other inflammatory problems. Frankincense relieves pain and inflammation by improving blood circulation and inhibiting damage to the hippocampus associated with learning and memory." (3)

Suddenly the lack of headaches after I found out I had the tumour might make sense. I had previously thought they had gone as my body no longer needed to tell me I had a serious problem that needed addressing. But the headaches went from me twitching with pain, barely able to move or walk and having to follow a pattern when I did, to almost nothing. Maybe it was the simple fact I brought the frankincense? Maybe the frankincense stopped me getting even worse? Did the frankincense help towards me leaving hospital so soon, and reduce the need for the head drain? Plus the headaches started up again a few days after I was told to stop all natural remedies I was taking at the pre-op assessment.

On Facebook I add my own following comment:

"Thank fuck mine wasn't cancerous ... But I wonder if the fact I was using frankincense oil orally as soon as found out I had a brain tumour meant that was why I didn't need the drain tube in head after op for long and why the headaches

had reduced after I found out ?? (I brought the oil almost as soon as I found out) And why they came back again over weekend before op as had been told to stop all alternatives ... ??

If this is true it could be a wonder drug... if it saved 3- 7 nights extra in hospital after op, and reduced the swelling ????"

A few days later I click on the references at the bottom on the Frankincense link and read this article:

"The anti-inflammatory effect of B. serrata has been studied in patients with brain tumors. An ethanolic extract of the gum resin of B. serrata contains boswellic acids. A study has shown that after the application of this preparation (which is called phytopharmacon H15) for a period of 7 days, a reduction of peritumoral brain edema by 22-48% was observed. In contrast to the cells of untreated patients, the cells of the treated tumor tissue showed no tendency to proliferate within 2 weeks.

A report on patients with malignant glioma showed that administering 3600 mg/day of Boswellia extract (60% boswellic acids), 7 days prior to surgery, caused decrease in the fluid around the tumor to an average of 30% in 8 of the 12 patients and the signs of brain damage decreased during the treatment.

Recently, a detailed study in patients with malignant cerebral tumors who were receiving radiotherapy plus certain amount of Boswellia extract showed that after radiotherapy, 75% reduction of cerebral edema was observed in 60% of the patients receiving Boswellia extract. The study also showed the ratio of tumor over volume decreased in these patients, suggesting the antitumor effect in addition to the anti-edema activity" (4)

Yes I know I had quite a lot of fluid on my neck after surgery, but it seemed to arrive and stay there from after the surgery, not later on. My fluid drain tube was clipped and removed around 24 hours after surgery when most people need them for several days. I know they clipped it mainly as I was touching near the area, but they said they couldn't have removed it if I still had lots of fluid, which was why it was clipped and not just removed to start with. Could this have still been some effect from the frankincense I had been taking for the few weeks before surgery?

And with the neck swelling after- I hadn't been taking frankincense at all after the surgery- I wasn't really up to taking lots of anything - it was hard enough to get food at times! My alternative health advisor was me, and I wasn't up to much more than the basics and didn't want to add anything into me that could somehow interfere with the healing and so just focussed on my homeopathy. It was only around the time I went back to check the fluid on my neck at 3 weeks after surgery and realised I needed to try and get this improving – as well as being given the all clear from needing any further medication , that I started using frankincense again. Although this time I only used it in an oil burner or rubbed it directly on my neck. Could this be what caused the neck swelling to finally disappear relatively quickly?

Chapter 31 - Realisations

21st March. Mum is here and we are outside trying to tidy the garden up. After a while I walk into Dave's office/shed and go to step back out the door, somehow slightly kick my foot on the doorstep and slip onto the doormat outside (I am sure my coordination is still not the best) but with that my shoe gives way (I had some old ballet style shoes on) and my ankle rolls over onto itself – at the same time I get a huge pain in the side of my foot. I yell and hobble inside to cover my already blackening foot with Arnica cream and get some ice. I have a huge lump on the side of it already. A couple of hours later and the bruise and swelling is horrendous, plus I have looked online and yes you can break your 5th metatarsal while twisting your ankle. I am sure it's broken- not that I have ever broken a bone in my life to compare. So we go to the local walk in clinic, get an x-ray which confirms I have broken it, get given a boot and crutches and sent home to rest.

But I don't like the crutches- they seem to make the pain worse when I walk with them as when my foot hits the floor it feels worse, plus although I queried this with the nurse when I got them- when I walk with the boot on the pain seems worse than without using it...so even that night I take the boot off and hobble around, only when I need to, with 1 of the crutches as balance. That way it feels far more comfortable, and is more practical. Not to mention the boot has a curved base and I just start to feel wobbly again, and I cannot cope with that. Or, maybe I just don't like listening to doctors and would prefer listening to my body to tell me what's good?

22nd March. As I am stuck on the damn sofa again (I am still trying to not use the boot, and to only walk when I have to) I make the most of it and spend several days writing this book. Is the universe just telling me I needed to keep writing – as I haven't done much writing for a few weeks?

25th March. Posted on Facebook.

> *"Not sure if I am mad, stubborn or insane. Just carried*
> *laptop, a glass of water and cup of herbal tea upstairs*
> *barefooted.*
> *I can't wear the bloody boot thing walking upstairs - the*
> *base is too curved and wobbly and I just feel 'drunk' again*
> *like I did with tumour- and I don't want anything to remind*
> *me of that feeling again ever...*
> *Thankfully I am good at walking on my heels and sides of*
> *feet* ☺ *although I can stand on broken foot lightly without*
> *pain x"*

30th March.

> *"Still a strange lump on side of foot, but it's a more normal*
> *colour and shape now* ☺
> *Not sure what they will tell me at fracture clinic tomorrow,*
> *but I am walking around barefoot ok now without pain -*
> *though still walking slightly on side of foot."*

31st March. Today I see the doctor at the fracture clinic, it is somewhat annoying to be stuck back in clinics and hospitals- I just don't want to do it again and am in a somewhat sarcastic mood about the whole thing. We sit in a cubicle and wait for the doctor and I feel rather like I have been a 'patient' all year- a burden. When the consultant arrives I tell him I ditched the crutches after a few days, I am barely wearing the boot- but do so when my foot or leg starts hurting as I have been walking too much with a 'twisted over' ankle so I don't put weight on the outside of the foot where I broke the bone. That I only wear it for a short time when my leg hurts, if I need to do something like put shopping away or if I might drop something on it. Oh and the boot is not thin enough for my leg...it only feels comfortable if I put a really thick thigh length sock on and fold it over a few times around my ankle. I am expecting to be told off that I should be wearing the boot all day, but no he says that is great, and to continue doing what I am doing as that way I will get less problems afterwards from lack of muscles etc that have been immobilised when the boot is on. Brilliant! I'm getting better at listening to myself and my body then!?

> "Hmm just realised I am walking on foot ok. 10 days isn't bad eh?! ❤"

The next few days I keep sitting in the garden contemplating how to change what is a sloped grass bank, into what I now imagine as a double layered flowerbed. Then I keep thinking I have a broken foot and will have to wait... but by 4th April I have realised I can walk the dog for a short distance at the park and can again fit normal trainers on loosely - so I start digging in the garden, even if much of it is sitting down and digging with a trowel.

6th April. Posted on Facebook.

> "Thank you everyone for my birthday wishes ❤
> Spent the day in the garden removing the sloped bank of grass and making raised flowerbeds instead. Doing it slightly slower than many -but have been there all day in the (unforcast) sun (even with broken foot!)
> Slightly knackered now... ☺
> But totally appreciating the difference from last year when I was barely able to move even a pot without my head pounding insanely as I bent down or thinking I would fall over with the dizziness."

9th April. When I am digging the soil, I keep seeing a robin who seems to be waiting for me to throw him some worms. But this robin doesn't look like a normal robin, he has barely any redness on his chest and his head just looks like he is missing feathers or is covered in scabs or white patches... he either has some disease or had a very close encounter with a cat? In fact if he didn't act like a robin I wouldn't really be sure he was one. However, whatever the reason is for his scars 'scabby robin' is just continuing to do what he has to - which I assume is feed babies - and he is in my garden for days, waiting for me to feed him the worms and grubs that I dig out.

I take a picture of him and see if anyone on my Facebook has any ideas on why he looks so bad... they don't, but also assume he must still have a nest as he is constantly eating!

> *"He is eating the worms I have been digging...lots of them! and sitting about 1m away (but not when I have a camera)"*

As I am watching him again I suddenly feel this, like he was sent here for a reason:

> *"I'm sure his head and neck has scabs on it so maybe he is 'my' robin. A slightly beaten up around the head with a few scars and war wounds, but alive, robin - just to make me smile ☺"*

... the day after this realisation, scabby robin disappears...

By the 12th of April (apart from the fact Dave and the family helped lift the bags of soil through to the front of the house) I have filed 60 bags of soil, put in 2 layers of 12 inch high wooden edge borders, filled them with the soil from the slope, added in a few slabs and slate as a pathway, moved the existing slabs around and extended the slate and pathway already there as well as planted some existing plants I had in the gaps. All with a broken foot! I fully appreciate that I am able to do this, it might be slow and I mainly use a trowel, but I have done it. I now have a garden with a flowerbed and flowers and not just a slippery, messy sloping grassed bank.

24th April. We go back to the caravan for the first time this year, and since my leaving rather abruptly last July. It is a little cold at night, even the dog seems cold! But we work out how to keep the caravan warm enough at night after a couple of days. This time I don't feel as shattered, I manage most days a reasonable walk to the beach or walk round the local ruins of a Roman castle, and the weather is actually quite warm and sunny by day. And I feel calmer.

At some point I decide to stay at the caravan while Dave and Roan are fishing and I look online and read this:

> *"Humans may be hard-wired to feel at peace in the countryside and confused in cities – even if they were born and raised in an urban area.*
> *According to preliminary results of a study by scientists at Exeter University, an area of the brain associated with being in a calm, meditative state lit up when people were shown pictures of rural settings. But images of urban environments resulted in a significant delay in reaction, before a part of the brain involved in processing visual complexity swung into action as the viewer tried to work out what they were seeing.*
> *The study, which used an MRI scanner to monitor brain activity, adds to a growing body of evidence that natural environments are good for humans, affecting mental and physical health and even levels of aggression.*
> *When looking at urban environments the brain is doing a lot of processing because it doesn't know what this environment is," he said. "The brain doesn't have an immediate natural response to it, so it has to get busy. Part of the brain that deals with visual complexity lights up: 'What is this that I'm looking at?' Even if you have lived in a city all your life, it*

seems your brain doesn't quite know what to do with this information and has to do visual processing," he said. Rural images produced a "much quieter" response in a "completely different part of the brain", he added. "There's much less activity. It seems to be in the limbic system, a much older, evolutionarily, part of the brain that we share with monkeys and primates." (5)

This makes so much sense to me, as a few months after brain surgery the desire to move to somewhere quiet was off the scale. I felt I <u>needed</u> it to heal, that surburbia was too much for me, and the few times I went into London it was almost physically hurting me at the end- I just wanted to go home. But I guess that if your brain had been through something traumatic, your body is healing and your reactions are still all slower than normal, then it would crave the simple. And this study shows that the countryside is a human default setting – it is wired for a natural calmness and tranquillity. Maybe that is why my brain was screaming for a rural life for so many months after? It knew what it needed to heal...

I continue looking online about the cerebellum I find this written in an article 'What does the Cerebellum really do?'

"Some years ago there was a report of an interesting deficit in a patient with massive right cerebellar hemisphere damage. When given the task of finding an appropriate verb for a noun that the experimenter recited, the patient made a number of inappropriate responses. If I were to say "car", you might respond "drive"; the patient made some peculiar and somewhat inappropriate responses. The logic seemed clear. The right hemisphere of the cerebellum projects to left cerebral cortex by way of the thalamus. In the patient, the cortical language area would be deprived of its input from the cerebellum, so there is a resultant deficit in word finding." (6)

This is me. I know I am frequently saying totally the wrong word, often similar but still wrong. I say necklace when I am talking about a bracelet, 'pass me the cup' when I mean a plate, or even a taxi when talking about a funeral procession car! I am far worse when I have to give directions, instructions or do something quickly, but I can still say totally the wrong word when I am at home and have not long woken up. When I look back I have been a bit like this for years- maybe not as much that others noticed, but I felt I was saying the wrong words far too often. This might all make more sense now.

> *"There are deficits in finger use in patients with cerebellar lesions. I would therefore argue that the cerebellum is related to skilled use of the fingers and accurate direction of the eyes."* (6)

Yes. I know I couldn't even colour in a kids colouring book for several months after my operation, my fingers couldn't keep the pen within the lines- it is only recently that at times I am able to colour in things for a short while, although even then if I look at something close for too long my eyes seem to blur up and I have to stop. The opticians say my eyes are fine, but I don't know if it is the damage from having the tumour or just getting older and going long sighted? Plus I cannot hold something in my hand and turn it very well, such as turning a key while carrying things, or twisting wire around a garden plant. This also accounts for the problem of not being able to type and control my fingers.

21ˢᵗ May. Posted on Facebook.
> *"1's again* ☺
> *Finally on way home after a gig* ❤*"*

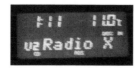

It's funny as I had a great evening. I had been relaxed and trusting despite being back in that pub where I first realised I was ill as I couldn't walk the stairs properly. I have been smiling to myself this evening that so much has changed in the 1 year since my operation- it is very much on my mind this week. Dave stops off for the shops on the way home and I am smiling listening to a song- and then see this. My 1's are here seemingly every time I am happy.

I have also been chasing up with Mr Jones' secretary at St George's, I had sent an email with various questions on it that I would like answered- and she gets back to me that they have booked me an appointment with him for August. It seems this year I am meant to wait. Learn patience.

14th July. The health ombudsman calls me. It feels they are digging for my thoughts and so I just listen. There is a new person taken over my case and they want to discuss the outcome of what they have decided so far...

That they will uphold my case against the G.P surgery that they should have removed my staples and should have done more to accommodate my needs, but at the moment- they are still writing the provisional report- they do not agree that the practice neglected their duty in failing to diagnose me. The woman seems to go silent and asks what I think. Well that's ridiculous as how can you say that if they admitted themselves they messed up by having a significant events analysis meeting? And what about their story that the doctor only offered me diazepam as the neck x-rays were showing muscle spasm- but I had not even had the x-ray yet. I told them I had many of what I now know are brain tumour symptoms and yet I wasn't even allowed a referral. How do I complain against your view as I am NOT happy with this as an answer? The doctors could have killed me from their neglect. The woman seems quiet and says she understands and will put a letter in the post to me with their findings, and that yes I can complain against the provisional report. I say I will be.

17th July. We are back in the caravan in Norfolk for a week's break. Today is our 20th Anniversary and despite the fact it not supposed to be good weather this week- it is sunny. Gorgeous blue skies. We decide to go to the beach. Sitting behind a windbreak and even the English weather is lovely and it feels we could be abroad, there is sand all around and the waves are sounding quieter than normal. I am lying down sunbathing, relaxing and healing, and as I look at the sky, what seems a small distance around the sun there is half a rainbow circle visible in the blue. It seems like the planet wants to celebrate with us too. I'm not sure if it's celebrating 20 years, or celebrating that we both feel different now. That this year has changed us both for the better? Telling us that you can have rainbows and glorious sun -without the rain.

End of July 2017. I am proof reading what I have written so far in this book and I re-read the information Tina sent me back in April last year. Suddenly these parts take on a new meaning:

> *"It was very clear instantly to me that Archangel Raphael is giving you the message that prayers do work, that prayers to God and the angels will be heard and will be answered by your recovery."*

Reading this again, I just smile. They truly did – I left hospital in 48 hours!!

> *"Have you met a new partner recently? Or are you in a relationship that could be leading to marriage? I ask because this Knight of Water card can also mean falling in love or wedding proposals. In your near future you are going to feel*

like moving on to something new, to something more meaningful because you will have grown both emotionally and spiritually. That could refer to a relationship or to your work.

Yes. Dave and I have totally changed, our relationship has changed- it has grown massively in the last few months. We both accept each other as we are more now. This year was our 20th anniversary and somehow things felt totally different to what they have before. I felt we had something to celebrate. I finally feel he gets me, that he is here for me 100%, that maybe I am not as weak as he thought, or that my health consciousness is not just a total waste of time- as he saw me getting myself better. That he understands that I don't need to drink or do anything that I don't want to do, and need to be true to me despite what others may say or think. Even though I have always been stubborn and done what I want, I still often worried what others thought. Now I really feel that's its 100% ok to be me. It is ok to let others know I am sad, or struggling, or tired or insanely happy. I cried every day for probably six months- and no one hates me for it. (Although if they do, I really don't care- it is their issue, not mine.) In fact it was liberating. I feel I let all the shock of finding I had a tumour and dealing with it, along with all the sadness I had bottled up over 42 years - and now they are gone. I feel he even understands the cause behind most of the things that we argue or disagree about and why they are happening. Yes we have both grown emotionally and spiritually.

Chapter 32 - Lessons of a Brain Tumour

August 2017. Written in journal. Again using my left hand for automatic writing, and now holding the hole in my head for direct access, asking the question: "What do I write in my book for the chapter- what I have learnt this last year or so?"

> *"Angels love you.*
>
> *They want you to see your true power within. To feel that strength inside. That you can perform miracles, if you just <u>listen</u> for the answer, in the peace.*
>
> *Not with your busy, thinking mind, but the part that just 'knows'.*
>
> *Listen, listen to your quiet mind, or your body will just give you the 'tools' to force you to hear.*
>
> *Follow your joy, follow your bliss. They are not in material possessions, they are in your thoughts, in your mind, in your heart, in your dreams. These will give you more strength than any object can.*
>
> *Always be true to you and we will be there supporting you 100% of the way.*
>
> *It's when you don't listen to yourself and die inside that we can't help you anymore. You have to prove you can be true to <u>you</u> again before we can intervene.*
>
> *But when you are true, when you listen to your inner self, no matter how hard things can be on the surface, we will always be supporting you.*

Sometimes you have to have hit that rock bottom to let go enough & to trust us to help. Otherwise you are stuck in that situation where your thoughts change the event. When you are at the bottom, you have no other way- you have exhausted all your rational thought. They haven't worked- so now you die or trust.

Love & trust is it all. The power to change worlds, the power to create miracles... or the power to get you out of hospital in 2 days!

You know. You learnt your lessons. Your world has changed.

Now it's over to others to do the same...

Lesson 1. Listen to yourself. You know.

Lesson 2. Know when to let go. (& trust you will be held by us and others)

Lesson 3. Tell us what you need, we cannot help without that.

Lesson 4. Everyone has this power in them, you are nothing special. (Although knowing this is pretty special enough! ☺)

Lesson 5. You can either:
  Feel love or hate.
  Feel strength or pain.
  Feel whole or broken.
  - *You always have the choice which option you pick.*

Lesson 6. Trust in magic – some things aren't possible, but they still happen.

Lesson 7. Let go of the past. You are not who you were yesterday.

Lesson 8. If you hold onto your past it literally does your head in. Let go. Be Free. Or you only hurt yourself.

Lesson 9. Life ever only gives you lemons to force you into that what you need to do. It gives you the bad so you have to change direction when you haven't been listening.

Lesson 10. You could be alive 3 minutes, 3 years or 3 decades & your joy can be the same amount.

Lesson 11. You <u>have</u> to find your joy. (If you want to keep alive)

Lesson 12. All of us are born with innate healing power, you have experienced that.

Lesson 13. You can directly influence your health, by your mood.

Lesson 14. Animals don't mope that they only have 3 legs left, they just get on with it with what they have.

Lesson 15. You only die when you lose hope.

Lesson 16. The joy is never the external circumstances, it's all within your mind.

Lesson 17. Be thankful for everything.

Lesson 18. Love, love & love a bit more. (The unconditional kind, not the 'I love you as you are pretty' kind)

Lesson 19.
    If someone is sad – love them.
    If someone is angry – love them.
    If someone is ill – love them. (& see them healed)
    If someone is hateful – love them.
    If someone is violent – love them.
    -   It's the only way things will change"

Lesson 20. Change is within us all, whenever we need it. Once we acknowledge what we need, and more importantly, what we need to let go of.
You just need to believe, trust and take small daily steps in the direction you are going.
We will support you all the way – you just have to ask."

I wish I could change the world, but the only part I can change is me and for others to understand that love too and change themselves. I believe that if we are all true to ourselves, question ourselves and don't just follow what we have always known or been told, that slowly we change things that we are not happy with and then peace and love can be possible.

I look back at the 'me' that started writing this book and I know I am now a different person inside to the one I have been for the last 43 years. I had read so, so many self-help books, people who had techniques and theories as to how their life had changed and how if you followed their steps and understood it, told you yours would to. Yes I often understood what they meant, but I didn't really feel it. It wasn't inside me. I didn't 'get' it. My life never changed, I never felt any more positive. I felt a failure at so many things. For some reason people don't praise you for bringing up 4 amazing children – as if the younger generation following their dreams and being happy doesn't count. I am not what the government would call a productive worthwhile citizen. I often felt it.

Yet having a brain tumour, a horrendous and terrifying experience, and surviving- even doing really well- changed everything. Knowing that there was something else bigger than just me in this world. Knowing that even in the darkest of torturous days in the hospital I could find that peace when I needed to, or find a technique that took my pain away from my head and took it into my tailbone. That I could go from extreme anxiety and panic to total calm and bliss in a few minutes – purely by changing my thoughts. Change how things felt totally. When I trusted. Oh and I have learnt patience, a tremendous amount of patience.

My brain simply forced me to slow down, to focus on that moment and not the past or future, and if I try to go too fast again- it still stops me. I break a foot, my back goes, or I just hit that wall of exhaustion.

It seems the more I trust the positive, the more I recover my coordination and realise that once again I am able to do the things even better than I could a couple of months ago, that I am not so shattered, that I feel so much healthier inside.

As I am contemplating this as I go to bed – after a very late evening finishing writing, and am feeling the gratitude of the lessons and change in me. This is a perfect example of what I see:

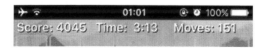

My angel numbers. The mirrored and repetitive numbers that help me when I am stuck or need to know something is here for us all. At 01.01 as I turn off my 'games phone' it also shows me 3.13 and 151.

Chapter 33 - Doesn't Everyone Hug their Brain Surgeon?

3rd August 2017. Today was the appointment with my brain surgeon to discuss the many question that have not actually been answered by anyone (but many of which after 15 months since surgery I think I know...)

I thought I was ok about this, that I was only seeing it as a positive experience. Finding the truth. But then this morning I got nervous. Maybe I won't like the answers? Maybe Mr Jones will think I am wasting his time? Maybe I still have risks?... Then to make me feel more stressed and I am wasting time, in the car on the way there Dave tells me he already knows most of the answers, as do I. So I tell Dave what I am thinking, that I want him to shut up about being negative as I feel I need to go. I need the answers and it is ok for me to expect answers and to see it as a positive experience.

I am fine until I walk into the hospital waiting room and then I can feel my stomach glugging and churning a little – a part of me still hates this place. (It is a hospital after all) As ever most of the patients in the waiting room are far older, but this time it's ok. I just want to go and ask them if they are alright too. I don't feel like I am 'unlucky' in having to be here. I am bloody lucky I am still here. I feel now that I know this is the final chapter. In having a tumour – as well as my book!

Dave and I are sitting on the chairs nearest to the consultation rooms and so we just see Mr Jones when he is almost standing behind us as we hear him say 'hello'. I ramble on about not really liking it much here and then say 'Oh no, not you or the staff, just waiting rooms in hospitals, just waiting, too many bad memories.'

So I sit down with my two pages of questions and say 'sorry for all these, but I just don't know some things and I need the answers'.

Basically – all the odd sensations I still have, the numbness, the feeling of a 'plate' in my head, the 'bruised pain' the sharp pains, the itching are all nerve damage. Yes it was the greater occipital nerve that was cut. No they didn't take any muscle away, but yes it has wasted quite a lot - as often happens. Yes the front hole is deep, but it's ok. Plus I still have a few more months for things to continue to improve, until about two years after the operation, which includes all the head nerve based issues as well as my coordination etc. After that recovery will really start to slow down.

I see my MRI and CT pictures from last year and I understand where the acrylic plate is better. I see I have a funny wrinkled looking area where the tumour was- as the cerebellum has moved back into the place where the tumour was. Then Mr Jones explains that the area looks good, but that it is like a grape being removed from jelly- it just doesn't go back perfectly. But my brain is back in the space it should be.

I laugh that on the MRI of the spine they have a picture clearly showing my bum cheeks, and it actually looks quite realistic! I say 'oh my god that's funny'. Mr Jones says something polite about not noticing. I reply 'I know, but I really don't care'. What I might have once been upset with or concerned about- it just doesn't matter. It's all ok.
Seeing the scan pictures of my head with and without the tumour, being told again that my tumour was really big for a hemangioblastoma, and being shown a quick sketch as to what they are often like... yet still I am really ok with it, all of it. I am curious now, thankful and extremely grateful ... and not tearful.

Mr Jones tells me that since my operation he has operated on 3 more patients with hemangioblastoma, which is a high number for him as there are only about 40 a year in the whole of the U.K. Trust me to be different!

He says "You look well, really well, now. Even healthier than last August." I say "Thank you, I feel it." I know I am a different person to who I was last year, and it seems others can see this too.

And I get thanked for my Christmas card I sent, he says he remembered it as it was handmade, he barely gets any cards and that he appreciated it. Dave and I laugh and Dave says he was lucky to get a card, I agree that I think I only sent about five Christmas cards, so tell Mr Jones that he was one of the lucky few! I am silently thinking... 'What's a card? It can't express the gratitude really can it? Maybe the words did? I know I sent them from the heart. Or maybe it means more if hardly anyone sends one?'

I then tell him about the frankincense seemingly stopping my headaches before the surgery, and that they came back after I had to stop it (after the pre op appointment) and that there is info on frankincense being able to do this in medical sites as well as the alternative ones. He says he will look into it more as it sounds interesting!

Then I ask "Can I put your name in my book?", and explain that I like reading about things and when I found out I had the tumour I couldn't find a book that I thought would help me. So I am writing one. A positive one. Then smile and say "I am not rude about you!" He agrees that it is fine, that I am allowed my personal opinion anyway, "but please just don't call me any C, W or F words!" to which I laugh that I haven't- although have plenty of those words in there!

Dave tells him that we probably knew the answers he gave, but it just clarifies them and stops me stressing. Mr Jones agrees and says "It's really just best to forget about it" (and it will help break the response cycle in itching etc) I do another silly grin and agree. I know my weaknesses, and can laugh about them. I will just have to sit on my hands more! And also realise simultaneously that I am starting to forget about being a brain tumour patient. It is my history - I am now a brain tumour survivor.

So we get up to leave, and he says something like 'It's good to see you looking so well, so will you give me a hug then?' and so I hug the man who saved my life. Apparently hugging your brain surgeon is acceptable after all!

And then I cry.

Then as I am walking from the room I laugh at him saying "See, and now you've made me cry again- and I'd almost managed not to cry at you at all..." and smile and say "but thanks."

And that is it. I really feel that's it. Bad chapter in life is over. I can move on now as it's finished.

Writing and art, here I come...

Afterword

As I am writing this at the end of August 2017 I am still receiving letters from the health ombudsman and have their draft report – which I am not allowed to disclose!

But I know that I will have to keep 'battling' with my complaint with them, not just so I can get some compensation for the direct costs that we incurred from the doctors at Giggs Hill failing me, but that it will help many others in the long run. If it helps just one G.P recognise the symptoms of a brain tumour better, especially on someone that may have a cancerous tumour, these few weeks may well save their life. I feel that even if I don't get a penny from the ombudsman that this is the right thing to do. And we all need to help others more. I will update my website with details of the outcome in due course.

Acknowledgements

To Nicola. Thank you for my Gaia healings, the virtual healings and sending me so much strength before my operation. ♥

To Alison. Thank you for all my Bowen treatments. They helped my body relax so much, especially after surgery. ♥

To Anna. Thanks for the very best gift ever for someone having an operation on their head- the cuddly toy kept my head propped up straight for many a night- and often still does! ♥

To Marion. Thank you for your presence and helping me understand mine. ♥

To Cherry. Thank you for your brilliant proof reading skills ♥

About the Author

Jo Barlow is a Mum of four, living in Surburbia. She has been
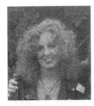reading self-help and spiritual books for several
years, yet only when having her own serious health
crisis did her own guidance kick in. IT'S ALL IN MY
HEAD is an enlightening memoir of both the worst
and best year of her life.

Resources.

Bowen Practitioner. Alison Rhys-Davies.
http://www.bowenarrow.co.uk

Craniosacral therapist. Paul Strode.
http://www.craniosacraltherapist.co.uk

Gaia Healing. Nicola Swan. http://www.nicolaswan.com

Journey Therapist. Marion Young. http://marionyoung.co.uk

Angel readings. Tina Wyatt.

Hollie Holden. http://www.hollieholden.me

Articles.

Mike Dooley TUT – Notes from the universe. http://www.tut.com

Teal Swan: The Spiritual Catalyst.
https://www.facebook.com/thespiritualcatalyst

'The Thing' full copy here:
http://www.rebellesociety.com/2016/06/03/estherdelaford-thing

German New Medicine. http://www.newmedicine.ca

Books.

The Brain's Way of Healing. By Norman Doidge.
http://www.normandoidge.com

Dying to be me. By Anita Moorjani. http://anitamoorjani.com

You can heal your life. By Louise Hay. http://www.louisehay.com

Getting into the Vortex CD. Abraham Hicks. http://www.abraham-hicks.com

UK Brain Tumour Support groups.

http://brainstrust.org.uk

https://www.thebraintumourcharity.org

References

(1) http://www.bbc.co.uk/news/health-31506317

(2) https://www.psychologytoday.com/blog/the-athletes-way/201405/neuroscientists-discover-the-roots-fear-evoked-freezing

(3) https://thetruthaboutcancer.com/preventing-brain-tumors/?utm_campaign&utm_medium=post&utm_source=facebook&utm_content=preventing-brain-tumors&utm_term=ttac-fans

(4) https://www.ncbi.nlm.nih.gov/pmc/articles/PMC3924999/

(5) http://www.independent.co.uk/news/science/human-brain-hard-wired-for-rural-tranquillity-8996368.html

(6) http://www.sciencedirect.com/science/article/pii/S096098220701785X

For products used, direct links to the resources above and further links.

Please see my website: www.JoBarlow.co.uk

Printed in Great Britain
by Amazon

43365081R00154